Diabetes & You

V.B. Blake

Introduction

There is much valuable information available on a wide variety of internet websites that will educate you on Diabetes: new treatments, what symptoms to look for, complications, lifestyle changes, and so on. It is not the intent of this small publication to educate you thoroughly on medical terminology or aspects of diabetes, which is a subject best left to the professional and highly trained individuals.

I hope this brief compilation of information will provide a general overview of diabetes with dietary suggestions that will guide you in making better nutritional and lifestyle choices.

Disclaimer

The material in this publication was sourced from various internet websites. It is intended for information purposes only and should not be used in place of consultation with a health care professional.

Table of Contents

What is Diabetes?

Diabetes is a disease in which blood glucose levels are above normal. Most of the food we eat is turned into glucose, or sugar, for our bodies to use for energy. Glucose is the preferred fuel for our body's cells and it's the only food our brain can use. The glucose floats along in the bloodstream until the the pancreas, an organ that lies near the stomach, makes a hormone called insulin that signals body cells to absorb the glucose. Once inside the cell, the glucose is either used as fuel to produce heat or energy or is stored as fat.

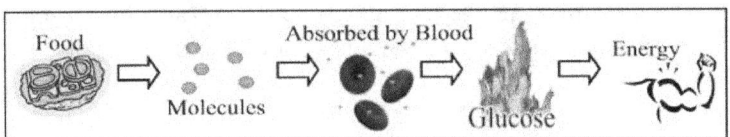

In a person with diabetes, the body either doesn't make enough insulin or can't use its own insulin as well as it should. When the glucose can't get into the cells, sugar accumulates in the blood and is later expelled in the urine. In other words, blood sugar rises while cells starve which can, potentially, harm certain organs and tissues.

In a healthy person, blood delivers glucose to provide the body with energy to perform all our daily activities.

- the liver converts the food a person eats into glucose which is then released into the bloodstream

- insulin is produced by the pancreas which helps digest food

- insulin allows glucose to move out of the blood into cells throughout the body where it is used for fuel.

Diabetes is a chronic condition and can last a life time. The goal of treating diabetes is to keep blood glucose levels as close to a normal range as possible which prevents the symptoms of diabetes and the long-term complications. Coping with diabetes is a lifelong challenge, so people with diabetes should not be afraid to speak with a doctor or pharmacist if they feel overwhelmed. Diabetes can cause serious health complications including heart disease, blindness, kidney failure, and lower-extremity amputations.

Part of a treatment plan for diabetes will involve learning about diabetes, how to manage it, and how to prevent complications. Your doctor, diabetes educator, or other health care professional will help you learn what you need to know so you are able to manage your diabetes as effectively as possible. Keep in mind that learning about diabetes and its treatment will take time. Involving family members or other people who are significant in your life can also help you manage your diabetes.

Types of Diabetes

There are three main types of diabetes.

Type 1 Diabetes

Type 1 diabetes is believed to be an autoimmune disease which causes the body's immune system to specifically attack the cells in the pancreas that produce insulin. More simply, the body stops producing insulin or produces too little insulin to regulate the blood glucose level.

- type 1 diabetes may run in families, however, genetic causes are much more common for type 2 diabetes, for example, a person with a parent, brother or sister with type 1 diabetes could develop the condition. Even though type 1 diabetes is difficult to predict, it is believed that genetics are the biggest indicators

- environmental factors, including common viral infections, such as mumps, have been known to trigger type 1 diabetes

- most common in people of non-Hispanic, Northern European descent (especially Finland and Sardinia), followed by African Americans, and Hispanic Americans. It is relatively rare in those of Asian descent

- type 1 diabetes is slightly more common in men than in women

- type 1 diabetes is typically diagnosed during childhood or adolescence. It used to be referred to as *juvenile-onset diabetes* or *insulin-dependent diabetes mellitus*

- type 1 diabetes can occur in an older individual due to destruction of the pancreas by alcohol, disease, or removal by surgery. It also results from progressive failure of the pancreatic beta cells, the only cell type that produces significant amounts of insulin

- people with type 1 diabetes require insulin treatment daily to sustain life.

Type 2 diabetes

Type 2 diabetes, formerly called *adult-onset diabetes* or *non-insulin-dependent diabetes*, is the most common form of diabetes and tends to run in families. People can develop type 2 diabetes at any age, even during childhood. This form of diabetes usually begins with *insulin resistance*, a condition in which fat, muscle, and liver cells do not use insulin properly. At first, the pancreas keeps up with the added demand by producing more insulin. In time, however, it loses the ability to secrete enough insulin in response to meals. Being overweight and inactive increases the chances of developing type 2 diabetes.

Gestational diabetes

Gestational diabetes is a type of diabetes that only pregnant women get and, if not treated, it can cause problems for mothers and babies. Gestational diabetes is caused by the hormones of pregnancy, or a shortage of insulin, and develops in 2% to 10% of all pregnancies but usually disappears when a pregnancy is over. Although this form of diabetes usually goes away after the baby is born, a woman who had gestational diabetes has a 35% to 60% chance of developing type 2 diabetes in the next 10–20 years.

Gestational diabetes occurs more frequently in African Americans, Hispanic/Latino Americans, American Indians, and people with a family history of diabetes than in other groups. Obesity is also associated with higher risk.

Pre-diabetes

Pre-diabetes is a condition in which blood glucose levels are higher than normal but not high enough for a diagnosis of diabetes. People with pre-diabetes are at increased risk for developing type 2 diabetes and for heart disease and stroke. The risk of getting pre-diabetes can be reduced with modest weight loss and moderate physical activity.

Type 3 diabetes

Recently a type 3 diabetes was discovered which is believed to be strongly linked to Alzheimer's Disease. When the brain produces lower than normal levels of brain insulin, the brain cells are deprived of insulin and they eventually die causing memory loss and other degenerative diseases.

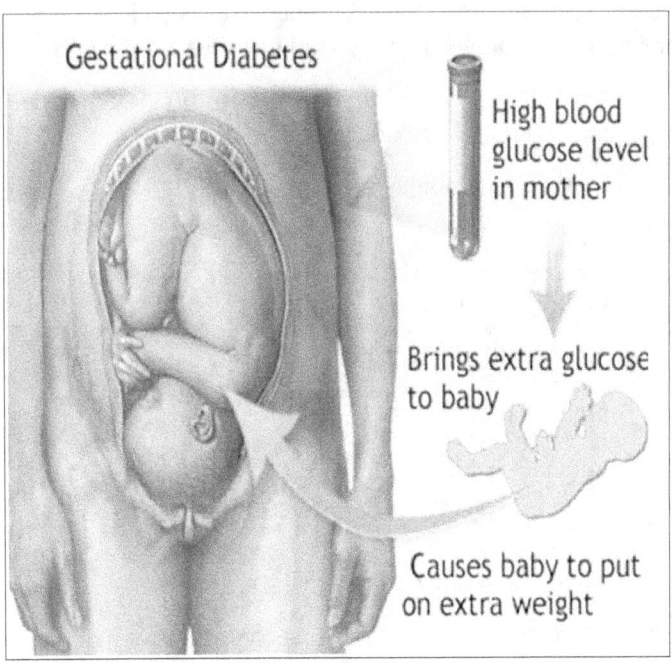

Gestational Diabetes

High blood glucose level in mother

Brings extra glucose to baby

Causes baby to put on extra weight

Risk factors

Risk factors are less well defined for type 1 diabetes than for type 2 diabetes, but autoimmune, genetic, and environmental factors are involved in developing this type of diabetes. A person who consumes excessive amounts of sugar is also likely to develop type 2 diabetes. Several genes have been identified, and more are under study, which may relate to the causes of type 2 diabetes.

Type 2 diabetes at risk include persons:

- high blood pressure

- high blood triglyceride (fat) levels

- gestational diabetes

- giving birth to a baby weighing more than 9 pounds

- high-fat diet

- high alcohol intake

- sedentary lifestyle

- obesity or being overweight

- ethnicity, particularly when a close relative had type 2 diabetes or gestational diabetes

- increasing age risk begins to rise significantly at about age 45 years and rises considerably after age 65 years

Symptoms

People who think they might have diabetes must visit a physician for diagnosis. Type 1 diabetes tends to come on rapidly with the classic symptoms of frequent urination, excessive thirst and fatigue while type 2 diabetes comes on more slowly, often over a course of years.

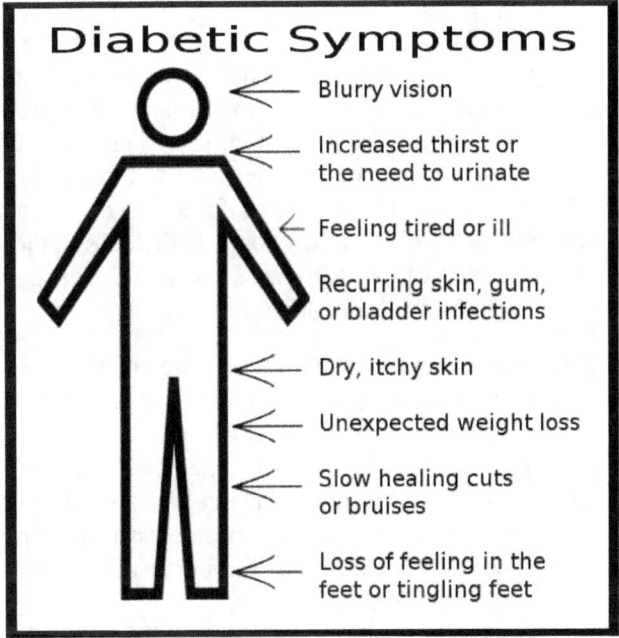

Type 1 diabetes

Type 1 diabetes is usually recognized in childhood or early adolescence, often in association with an illness (such as a virus or urinary tract infection) or injury. The extra stress can cause diabetic ketoacidosis. Symptoms of ketoacidosis include nausea and vomiting. Without treatment, ketoacidosis can lead to coma and death.

Type 2 diabetes

A person may have type 2 diabetes for many years without knowing it. If not treated, type 2 diabetes can lead to complications such as blindness, kidney failure, heart disease, and nerve damage. People with type 2 diabetes can develop *hyperglycemic hyperosmolar nonketotic syndrome.*

Common symptoms of both type 1 and type 2 diabetes:

- fatigue, constantly tired - in diabetes, glucose from the food we eat travels into the bloodstream where insulin is supposed to help it transition into the cells of our body. The cells use it to produce the energy we need to live. When the insulin isn't there or if the cells don't react to it any more, the glucose stays outside the cells in the bloodstream. The cells become energy starved causing fatigue and a tired, run down feeling.

- weight loss - people with diabetes are unable to process many of the calories in the foods they eat. This symptom is more noticeable with type 1 diabetes where the pancreas stop making insulin. When the cells aren't getting glucose the body desperately looks for an energy source which results in using muscle tissue and fat. Type 2 happens gradually with increasing insulin resistance so weight loss is not as noticeable.

- excessive thirst - a person with diabetes develops high blood sugar levels which overwhelms the kidney's ability to reabsorb the sugar. The kidney spills the over-abundance of sugar as excessive urination. The body tries to counteract this by encouraging more water consumption to dilute the high blood sugar back to normal levels and to compensate for the water lost by excessive urination.

- excessive urination - the body tries to rid extra sugar in the blood by excreting it in the urine. This can also lead to dehydration as a large amount of water is necessary to excrete the sugar. If insulin is non-existent or ineffective, the kidneys can't filter glucose back to the blood and become overwhelmed. They will try to draw the extra water out of the blood, in an effort to dilute the glucose, which keeps the bladder full and causing frequent urination.

- excessive eating - if the body is able, it will secrete more insulin in order to try to manage the excessive blood sugar levels. As one of the functions of insulin is to stimulate hunger, these higher insulin levels lead to increased hunger. However, despite increased caloric intake, the person may gain very little weight and may even lose weight.

- poor wound healing - high blood sugar levels prevent white blood cells from functioning normally. White blood cells defend the body against bacteria and also in cleaning up dead tissues and cells. When these cells do not function properly, wounds take much longer to heal and become infected more frequently. Long-standing diabetes is associated with thickening of blood vessels, which prevents good circulation including the delivery of enough oxygen and other nutrients to body tissues.

- infections - certain infections, such as frequent yeast infections of the genitals, skin infections, and frequent urinary tract infections, may result from suppression of the immune system by diabetes and by the presence of glucose in the tissues, which allows bacteria to grow. These infections can also be an indicator of poor blood sugar control in a person known to have diabetes.

- altered mental status - agitation, unexplained irritability, inattention, extreme lethargy, or confusion can all be signs of very high blood sugar, *ketoacidosis*, *hyperosmolar hyperglycemia nonketotic syndrome*, or *hypoglycemia*.

- blurry vision - blurry vision is not specific for diabetes but is frequently present with high blood sugar levels.

- tingling or numbness in the hands or feet - this symptom is called *neuropathy* and it occurs over time as high glucose in the blood damages the nervous system, particularly in hands and feet. It is a gradual onset with type 2 diabetes so people are often not aware they have it.

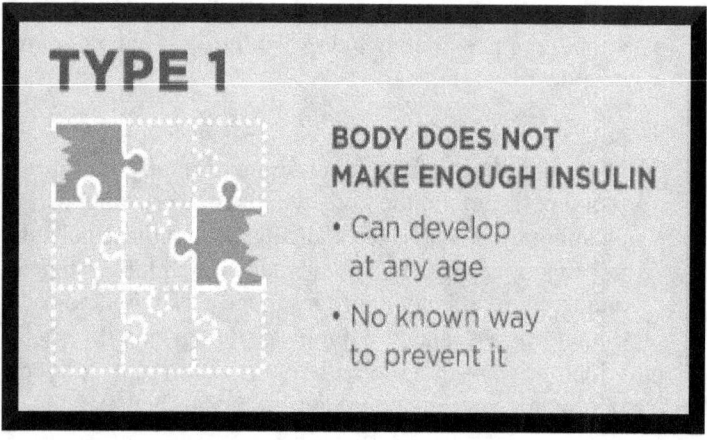

TYPE 1

BODY DOES NOT MAKE ENOUGH INSULIN

- Can develop at any age

- No known way to prevent it

How diabetes is diagnosed

Diabetes is diagnosed with simple blood tests or based on the results of an oral glucose tolerance test. With this test a person fasts and then is given a drink containing 75g of carbohydrate. The blood sugar is checked at fasting and two hours after drinking the solution.

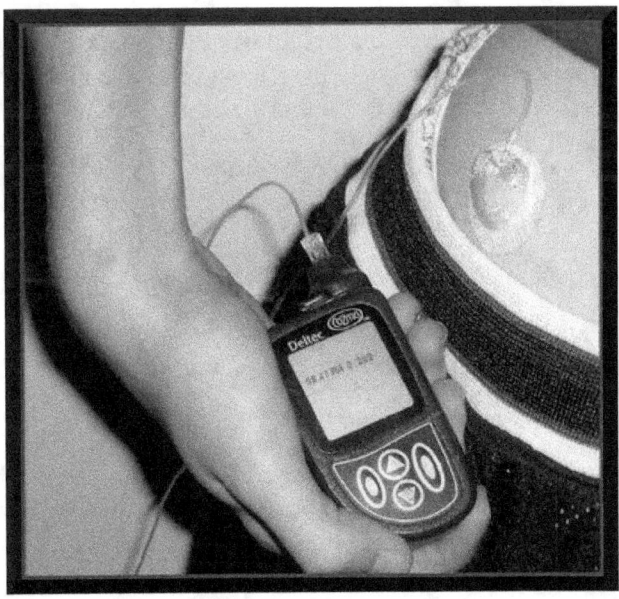

Treatment

People with diabetes must take responsibility for their day-to-day care and blood glucose levels must be closely monitored through frequent blood glucose testing. Healthy eating, physical activity, and insulin injections are the basic treatments for type 1 diabetes.

Healthy eating, physical activity, and blood glucose testing are the basic therapies for type 2 diabetes. In addition, many people with type 2 diabetes require oral medication, insulin, or both to control their blood glucose levels.

Working with a health care provider will assist in monitoring with diabetes control and help the patient learn to manage their diabetes. In addition, people with diabetes may see:

- endocrinologists, who may specialize in diabetes care

- ophthalmologists, for eye examinations

- podiatrists for routine foot care

- dietitians and diabetes educators who teach the skills needed for daily diabetes management

Why Self-Care is So Important

Daily self-care and treatment will help keep blood glucose, blood pressure, and cholesterol at an optimum range and help prevent other health problems that diabetes can cause over the years.

Following a daily regime can do a lot to prevent diabetes problems, such as:

- following a meal plan
- taking diabetes medications as prescribed
- be physically active
- checking blood glucose as recommended.

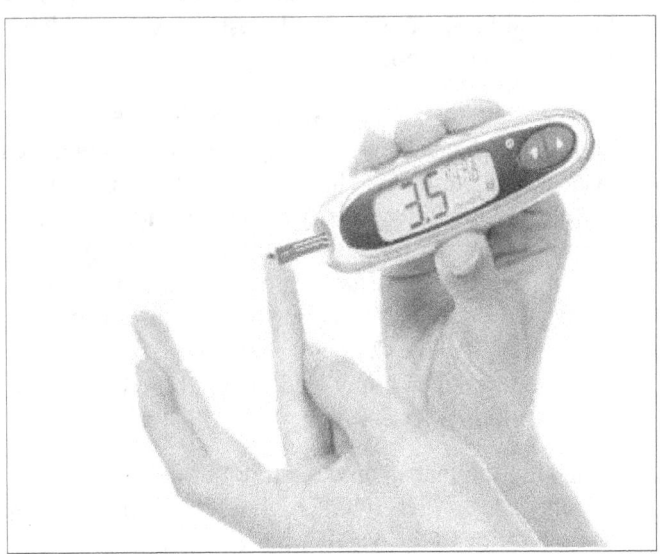

Diabetes and Your Heart and Blood Vessels

The biggest problem for people with diabetes is heart and blood vessel disease which can lead to heart attacks and strokes. It also causes poor blood flow to the legs and feet. At least once a year have a blood test to see how much cholesterol is in the blood and to check for heart and blood vessel disease.

- eat foods that are low in sodium. Sodium is an element found in table salt and in many foods in our diet. Health Canada recommends 1000 mg to 1500 mg per day. Sodium doesn't necessarily come from adding salt to food but rather from the sodium levels in highly processed foods; the amount of sodium in foods is indicated on food packages. Sodium is an essential nutrient and while the body needs some sodium to function, too much may lead to high blood pressure, heart or kidney disease

- keep blood glucose on track through frequent or daily monitoring as prescribed by your physician or health care provider. Glucose monitoring at home measures blood sugar at a particular moment. At least twice a year an A1C test, (*HbA1c, glycated hemoglobin or glycosylated hemoglobin*) should be undertaken which will determine the average blood glucose level over a longer period

- keep blood pressure at an optimum level. When blood pressure is high, it puts stress on the body which can cause damage to the heart, brain, kidneys, and eyes.

High blood glucose levels are a risk factor for high blood pressure as it can lead to hardening of the arteries.

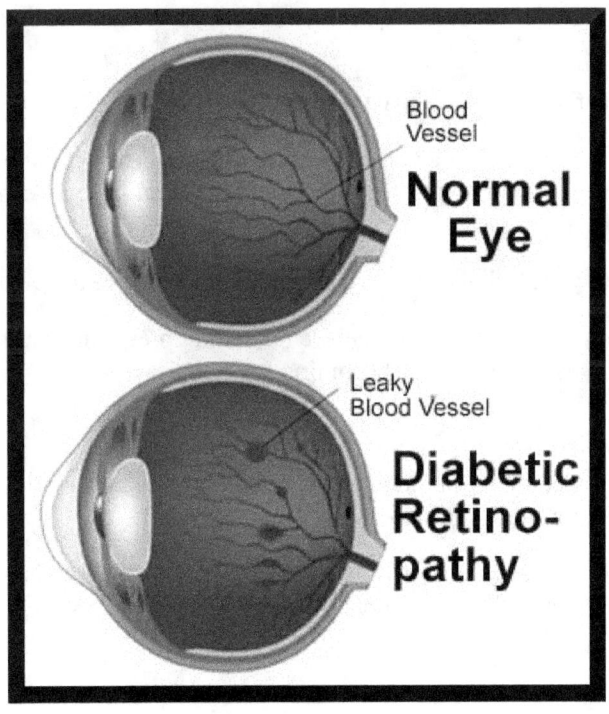

Diabetes and Your Eyes

High blood glucose can make the blood vessels in the eyes bleed which can lead to blindness. Keeping blood glucose and blood pressure as close to normal as possible can help in preventing vision problems. Yearly eye examinations may catch problems early.

Follow these tips to take care of your eyes:

- type 1 diabetes: have your eyes examined within 5 years of being diagnosed with diabetes. Then have an exam every year

- type 2 diabetes: have an eye exam every year

- have an eye exam before becoming pregnant or as soon as possible after becoming pregnant

- if you smoke, quit

- keep your blood glucose and blood pressure as close to normal as possible

- contact a doctor right away if you have blurry vision or are seeing dark spots, flashing lights, or rings around lights.

Diabetes and Your Kidneys

Kidneys help clean waste products from the blood and work to keep the right balance of sodium and fluid in the body. Twenty to forty percent of people with diabetes can develop a kidney disease called *diabetic nephronpathy* which, until its late stages, can be detected only by specific blood and urine tests. By the time symptoms develop the condition can be debilitating. See a doctor as quickly as possible in the event of bladder or kidney infections.

Signs of bladder or kidney infections are:

- cloudy or bloody urine

- pain or burning during urination

- having to urinate often or in a hurry

- back pain, chills, and fever are also signs of kidney infection.

Having the following tests, at least once a year, will ensure the kidneys are working well:

- a urine test for protein

- a blood test for *creatinine*, a waste product made by your body.

Diabetes and Your Nerves

Over time, high blood glucose can harm the nerves in the body. Nerve damage can cause loss the feeling in feet or to have painful, burning feet. Poor circulation as a result of blood vessel problems in legs can result in sores on feet that have trouble healing and might become infected. If the infection isn't treated it could lead to amputation. Nerve damage can also cause pain in legs, arms, or hands or cause problems with digesting food, going to the bathroom, or having sex.

Nerve damage can happen slowly and the person may not even realize there are nerve problems. Damaged nerves may stop sending messages, or may send messages slowly or at the wrong times. This damage is called *diabetic neuropathy* and approximately 50% of people with diabetes get it. Controlling blood sugar levels can help prevent nerve problems, or keep them from getting worse.

- numbness in hands, legs or feet

- shooting pains, burning or tingling

- nausea, vomiting, constipation or diarrhea

- problems with sexual function

- urinary problems

- dizziness when you change positions quickly.

You can prevent nerve problems to the feet by:

- keeping blood glucose and blood pressure as close to normal as possible

- limiting your intake of alcohol

- checking feet every day

- quit smoking

The World Health Organization predicts diabetes will become the seventh leading cause of death in the world by 2030. In 2012 diabetes was the direct cause of 1.5 million deaths.

Diabetes and Your Gums and Teeth

Diabetes can lead to infections in your gums and the bones that hold your teeth in place. Like all infections, gum infections can cause blood glucose to rise. Without treatment teeth may become loose and fall out. Sore, swollen, and red gums that bleed when you brush your teeth are a sign of a dental problem called *gingivitis*. Another problem, called *periodontitis*, happens when your gums shrink or pull away from your teeth.

There are a number of ways to help prevent infections:

- brush your teeth at least twice a day to prevent gum disease and tooth loss. Be sure to brush before you go to sleep and use a soft toothbrush and toothpaste with fluoride. To help keep bacteria from growing on your toothbrush, rinse it after each brushing and store it upright with the bristles at the top. Get a new toothbrush at least every 3 months

- besides brushing, you need to floss between your teeth each day to help remove *plaque*, a film that forms on teeth and can cause tooth problems. Flossing also helps keep your gums healthy. Your dentist or dental hygienist will help you choose a good method to remove plaque, such as dental floss, bridge cleaners, or water spray. If you're not sure of the right way to brush or floss, ask your dentist or dental hygienist for help

- get your teeth cleaned and checked at your dentist's office at least once every 6 months. See a dentist right away if you have trouble chewing or any signs of dental disease, including bad breath, a bad taste in your mouth, bleeding or sore gums, red or swollen gums, or sore or loose teeth

- plan dental visits so they don't change the times you take your insulin and meals. Don't skip a meal or diabetes medicine before your visit.

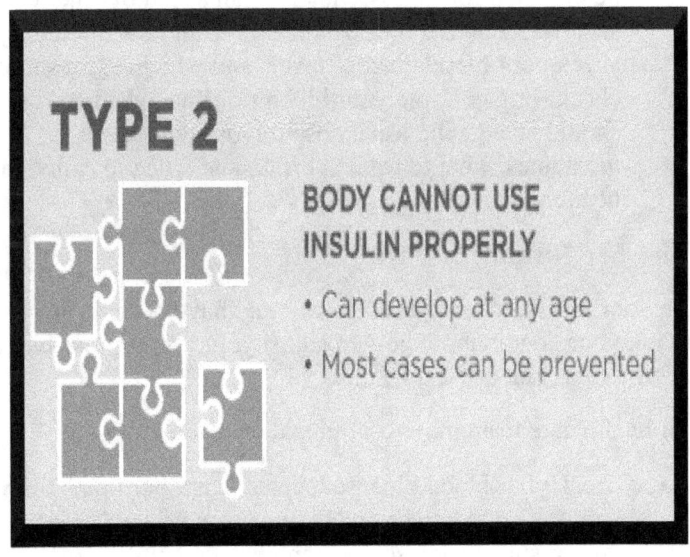

TYPE 2

BODY CANNOT USE INSULIN PROPERLY

- Can develop at any age
- Most cases can be prevented

Taking Care of Your Diabetes at Special Times

When You're Sick

Having a cold, the flu, or an infection can raise your blood glucose levels which can lead to serious health problems and even a coma.

- be prepared for illness. Make a plan ahead of time for sick days and ask your health care team how often to check your blood glucose levels and whether you should check for *ketones* in your blood or urine, whether you should change the usual dose of your diabetes medicines, what to eat and drink, and when to call your health care provider.

If You Use Insulin:

Take your insulin, even if you are sick and have been throwing up. Ask your doctor about how to adjust your insulin dose based on your blood glucose test results.

Your health care team may recommend the following:

- check your blood glucose level at least four times a day and write down the results in your record book. Keep your results handy so you can report results to your health care team

- keep taking your diabetes medicines, even if you're not able to eat

- drink at least 1 cup, or 8 ounces, of water or other calorie-free, caffeine-free liquid every hour while you're awake

If you can't eat the usual foods, try eating or drinking any of the following:

- juice

- saltine crackers

- dry toast

- soup

- broth or bouillon

- popsicles or sherbet

- regular, not sugar-free, gelatin

- milk

- yogurt

- regular, not sugar-free, soda

If You Don't Use Insulin:

Take your diabetes medicines, even if you are sick and have been throwing up.

Your health care provider may say you should call right away if:

- blood glucose levels are above 240 even though you've taken your diabetes medicines

- urine or blood *ketone* levels are above normal

- vomiting more than once

- diarrhea for more than 6 hours

- trouble breathing

- high fever

- you can't think clearly or you feel sleepier than usual

You should call your health care provider if you have questions about taking care of yourself.

At School or Work:

Take care of your diabetes when you're at school or at work:

- follow a meal plan

- take medicines and check blood glucose as usual

- tell teachers, friends, or close co-workers about the signs of low blood glucose - you may need their help if your blood glucose drops too low

- keep snacks nearby and carry some with you at all times to treat low blood glucose

- tell your company nurse or school nurse that you have diabetes.

Travelling Away From Home:

Though diabetes will certainly complicate your life it shouldn't rob you of your everyday pleasures. Travelling, for instance, will take extra preparation but planning ahead for any eventuality will make it less worrisome.

These travel tips can help you take care of yourself when you're away from home:

- follow your meal plan as much as possible when you eat out. Always carry a snack with you in case you have to wait to be served

- limit your drinking of beer, wine, or other alcoholic beverages. Ask your diabetes educator how much alcohol you can safely drink. Eat something when you drink to prevent low blood glucose

- avoid sitting for long periods. Get up and stretch whenever possible. If you are in a car, make regular stops to get up and walk around

- on a road trip plan ahead so that the timing of your insulin, meals, snacks and exercise doesn't change

- take twice as many supplies than you plan to use. You could be delayed or unable to find a drug store if you are travelling outside the country

- if you are crossing time zones your insulin schedules may need some adjustments. Talk to a diabetes team member about your travel plans

- carry a prescription for your medicines and syringes. It's not a bad idea to have a travel companion carrying duplicate copies

- if you're taking a long trip by car, check your blood glucose before driving. Stop and check your blood glucose every 2 hours. Always carry snacks like fruit, crackers, juice, or soft drinks in the car in case your blood glucose drops too low

- bring food for meals and snacks with you

- carry your diabetes medicines and your blood testing supplies with you. Never put them in your checked baggage

- take comfortable, well-fitting shoes on vacation. You'll probably be walking more than usual, so you should take good care of your feet

- if you're going to be away for a long time, ask your doctor for a written prescription for your diabetes medicines and the name of a doctor in the place you're going to visit

- don't count on buying extra supplies when you're travelling, especially if you're going to another country.

Different countries use different kinds of diabetes medicines

- consult with an airline for applicable international regulations

When There's an Emergency or Natural Disaster:

Everyone with diabetes should be prepared for emergencies and natural disasters, such as power outages or hurricanes. Consider storing three days worth of diabetes supplies. You may also want to have an extra glucagon emergency kit. All these items should be kept in an easy-to-identify container and stored in a location that is easy to get to in an emergency.

Examples of items for your Diabetes Emergency Kit:

- a minimum of two weeks worth of supplies and medications in a plastic storage bag

- packaged crackers and cheese/peanut butter

- flashlight, candles and matches

- extra glucose meter, extra insulin(s), glucagon, syringes, lancets, blood test strips, ketone test strips (blood or urine), alcohol wipes, insulin pump supplies, an insulated bag to keep insulin cool

- your diabetes medicines

- emergency glucose such as unopened glucose tablets

- non-diabetes medication such as anti-nausea and anti-diarrhea medication

- a list of all prescription numbers

- glucose tablets and other foods or drinks to treat low blood glucose

- antibiotic cream or ointment

- a copy of your medical information, including a list of your conditions, medicines, and recent lab test results

- phone numbers for the Canadian Red Cross and other disaster relief organizations

- emergency telephone numbers including that of your physician

- batteries for flashlights, meters, and pumps

- bottled water

- non-perishable foods such as canned goods, granola bars, and peanut butter - don't forget the can opener

- basic first aid kit

Check and update your kit at least twice a year.

When You're Planning a Pregnancy:

Keeping your blood glucose near normal before and during pregnancy helps protect both you and your baby. Even before you become pregnant your blood glucose should be close to the normal range. Consult your health care provider to discuss your insulin needs as they may change when you're pregnant.

- work with your health care team to get your blood glucose as close to the normal range as possible before you get pregnant

- see a doctor who has experience in taking care of pregnant women with diabetes

- don't smoke, drink alcohol, or use harmful drugs

- follow the meal plan you get from your dietitian

- have your eyes, heart and blood vessels, blood pressure, and kidneys checked. Your doctor should also check for nerve damage. Pregnancy can make some health problems worse.

Can diabetes be prevented?

Researchers are making progress in identifying the exact genetics and 'triggers' that predispose some individuals to develop type 1 diabetes, but prevention remains elusive. Thirty to sixty percent of type 2 diabetes can be prevented with lifestyle changes including a healthy diet and regular exercise.

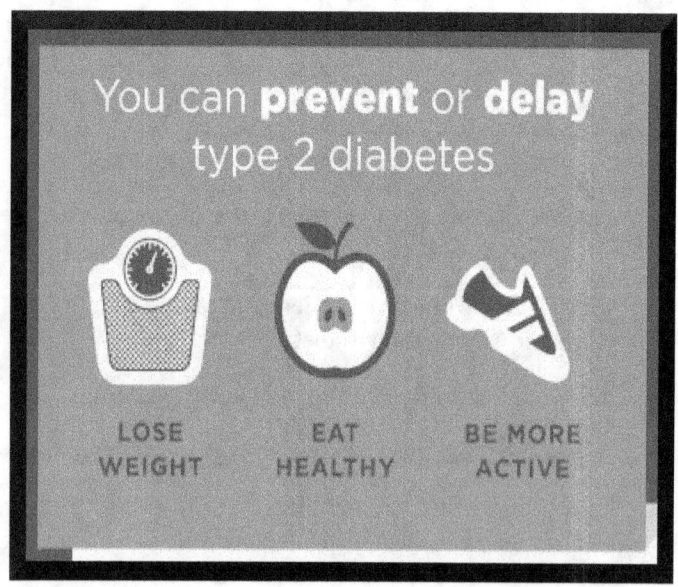

Can Diabetes be Cured?

No. Diabetes can be managed, but there is no cure for diabetes, yet. Any product that claims to be a miracle cure for diabetes is a fraud that could cheat you of time, money and most importantly, your health. Until researchers find a cure, the only safe way to manage diabetes is to follow the treatment program designed by your health care practitioner.

Several approaches to 'cure' diabetes are currently under investigation and include:

- pancreas transplantation

- islet cell transplantation (islet cells produce insulin)

- artificial pancreas development

- genetic manipulation (fat or muscle cells that don't normally make insulin have a human insulin gene inserted - then these 'pseudo' islet cells are transplanted into people with type 1 diabetes).

Diabetes Prognosis

Diabetes is a leading cause of death in all industrialized nations. Overall, the risk of premature death of people with diabetes is twice that of people who do not have diabetes. Prognosis depends on the type of diabetes, degree of blood sugar control, and development of complications.

Type 1 diabetes

About 15% of people with type 1 diabetes die before age forty, which is about twenty times the rate of that age group in the general population. The most common causes of death are diabetic *ketoacidosis*, kidney failure, and heart disease. Maintaining optimum blood sugar levels has been proven to prevent, slow the progression of, and even improve complications of type 1 diabetes.

Type 2 diabetes

The life expectancy of people who are diagnosed with type 2 diabetes in their forties decreases by five to ten years because of the disease. Heart disease is the leading cause of death for people with type 2 diabetes. Excellent *glycemic* control, tight blood pressure control, and keeping the 'bad' cholesterol (LDL) level at the recommended level and the 'good' (HDL) cholesterol as high as possible.

Complications

Both type 1 and type 2 diabetes ultimately leads to high blood sugar levels, a condition called hyperglycemia. Over a long period of time, hyperglycemia damages the retina of the eye, the blood vessels of the kidneys, the nerves, and other blood vessels and increases the risk of heart disease and kidney disease.

- damage to the retina from diabetes is a leading cause of blindness

- damage to the kidneys from diabetes is a leading cause of kidney failure

- damage to the nerves from diabetes is a leading cause of foot wounds and ulcers, which often leads to foot and leg amputations

- damage to the nerves in the autonomic nervous system can lead to paralysis of the stomach, chronic diarrhea, and an inability to control heart rate and blood pressure when sitting, standing, or walking

- diabetes accelerates *atherosclerosis*, which can lead to blockages or a *clot*. Such changes can then lead to heart attack, stroke, and decreased circulation in the arms and legs

- diabetes can lead to elevated blood pressure, high levels of cholesterol and triglycerides.

Diabetes can contribute to a number of short-lived medical problems, for example:

- infections are of particular concern for diabetics as high blood sugar levels can weaken the patient's immune system defences. Some diabetes-related health issues, such as nerve damage and reduced blood flow to the extremities, increase the body's vulnerability to infection

- *hypoglycemia* or low blood sugar, occurs intermittently in most people with diabetes. It can result from taking too much diabetes medication or insulin (sometimes called an insulin reaction), missing a meal, exercising more than usual, drinking too much alcohol, or taking certain medications for other conditions. It is very important to recognize *hypoglycemia* and be prepared to treat it at all times. Headache, feeling dizzy, poor concentration, tremor of the hands, and sweating are common symptoms of *hypoglycemia*. A person can faint or have a seizure if blood sugar level become too low

- diabetic *ketoacidosis* is a serious condition in which uncontrolled *hyperglycemia* (usually due to complete lack of insulin or a relative deficiency of insulin) over time creates a build up of *ketones* (acidic waste products) in the blood. High levels of *ketones* can be very harmful. This typically happens to people with type 1 diabetes who do not have good blood glucose control. Diabetic *ketoacidosis* can be brought on by infection, stress, trauma, missing medications like insulin, or medical emergencies such as a stroke and heart attack

- *hyperosmolar hyperglycemic nonketotic syndrome* is a serious condition in which the blood sugar level gets very high. The body tries to get rid of the excess blood sugar by eliminating it in the urine. This increases the amount of urine significantly, and often leads to dehydration so severe that it can cause seizures, coma, and even death. This syndrome typically occurs in

people with type 2 diabetes who are not controlling their
blood sugar levels, who have become dehydrated, or
who have stress, injury, stroke, or are taking certain
medications, like steroids.

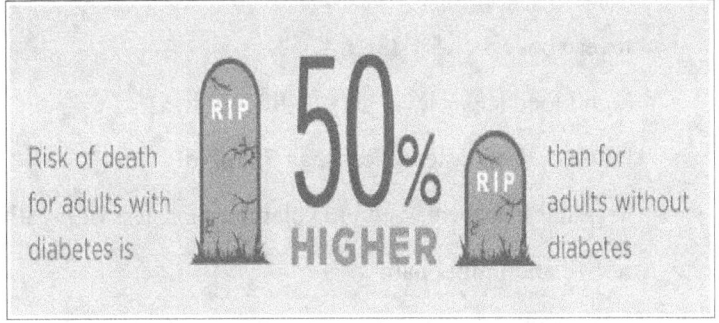

Risk of death for adults with diabetes is **50%** **HIGHER** than for adults without diabetes

When to Seek Medical Care

If a person has diabetes and experiences any of the following, call a health care professional:

- nausea or vomiting

- fever above 101.5°F (38.6°C)

- high blood sugar level above 400 mg/dL

- low blood sugar level less than 70 mg/dL

- irregular heartbeats and unexplained shortness of breath

- severe abdominal pain

- injury to the foot or leg, no matter how minor

- any cut penetrating all the layers of skin, especially on the legs

- chest pain, particularly in the middle or on the left side

Glucose Monitoring

It is essential for you to self-monitor blood glucose levels which is a key to taking charge of diabetes. The number of times you should test your blood glucose will be based on the type of diabetes you have and your diabetes treatment program. Frequent measurement of blood glucose levels, at different times of the day, is the best way to know whether blood glucose levels are in the target range.

Tests are easily done by pricking a finger and placing a drop of blood on a special coated strip which 'reads' your blood glucose. Many people use an electronic meter to get this reading most of which now have 'memory' that stores the number of blood glucose tests along with the time and date they were taken. Some even allow for graphs and charts of the results to be created when the monitor is connected to a computer. If your meter does not have a 'memory' it is important that you keep a log book or record sheet of each glucose reading indicating date and time you took it.

A blood test done in the laboratory called the *glycosylated hemoglobin test,* or A1c test, allows your doctor to see the average of blood glucose values over the last 3 months. This is a good indication of how well your blood glucose has been in control overall and allows your doctor to manage your diabetes more effectively.

What affects blood glucose levels?

Sometimes, no matter how hard you try to keep your blood glucose in your target range, it will be too high or too low. Blood glucose that's too high or too low can make you feel sick. Ask your health care provider how to handle these emergencies.

High blood glucose

High blood glucose means you don't have enough insulin in your body. High blood glucose, also called *hyperglycemia*, can happen if you miss taking your diabetes medicines, eat too much, or don't get enough exercise. Sometimes, the medicines you take for other problems can cause high blood glucose.

Some people with type 2 diabetes may not feel the signs of high blood glucose until their blood glucose is higher than 300. People with blood glucose higher than 300 are more likely to have dehydration which can become a serious problem if not treated right away.

Your blood glucose is more likely to go up when you're sick - for example, when you have the flu or an infection. You'll need to take special care of yourself during these times.

Signs of High Blood Glucose

Some common signs of high blood glucose are having a dry mouth, being thirsty, and urinating often. Other signs include feeling tired, thirst, frequent urination, blurred vision, dry or itchy skin, hunger, unexplained weight loss, cuts that won't heal, numbness or tingling in hands and feet. If your glucose is very high, you may have stomach pain, feel sick to your stomach, or even throw up. This is an emergency and you need to go to the hospital right away.

Sometimes there are no symptoms when your blood glucose is high. The only way you can be sure what your blood glucose is, is to check it. If you have any signs that your blood glucose is high, check your blood. In your logbook or on your record sheet, write down your glucose reading and the time you did the test. If your glucose is high think about what could have caused it to go up. If you think you know of something, write this down beside your glucose reading.

High glucose levels can be caused by:

- Carbohydrates - An increase in the amount and/or type of carbohydrates you eat. Most foods, except fats and meats, contain carbohydrates. When you eat foods that have a high concentration of carbohydrates per serving, or you have an increased amount of your usual foods, your blood glucose will rise

- Glucose released by the liver overnight - Your body requires glucose 24 hours a day, seven days a week. Your liver stores glucose and releases it during the night. With type 2 diabetes, your liver can sometimes release too much glucose which explains why your glucose may be higher in the morning than before you went to bed - even when you've had nothing to eat

- Illness - An illness can pose special problems for people who have diabetes. Illness is a stress on your body that can cause your blood glucose levels to go up. Even a minor illness such as a cold, flu or infection can raise your blood glucose level

- Stress - Emotional stress caused by excitement, anger, worry and fear can cause an increase in blood glucose

- Not enough medication - When you have less medication than normal, for example, you miss a dose, or the medication you are taking is not effective enough, blood glucose levels will rise

Low Blood Glucose

Low blood glucose, also called *hypoglycemia*, happens if your blood glucose drops too low. It can come on fast. Low blood glucose can be caused by taking too much diabetes medicine, missing a meal, delaying a meal, exercising more than usual, or drinking alcoholic beverages. Sometimes, medicines you take for other health problems can cause blood glucose to drop.

Low blood glucose can make you feel weak, confused, irritable, hungry, or tired. You may sweat a lot or get a headache. You may feel shaky. If your blood glucose drops lower, you could pass out or have a seizure.

If you have any of these symptoms, check your blood glucose. If the level is below 70, have one of the following right away:

- 3 or 4 glucose tablets

- 1 serving of glucose gel - the amount equal to 15 grams of carbohydrate

- 1/2 cup, or 4 ounces, of any fruit juice

- 1/2 cup, or 4 ounces, of a regular, not diet, drink

- 1 cup, or 8 ounces, of milk

- 5 or 6 pieces of hard candy

- 1 tablespoon of sugar or honey

After 15 minutes, check your blood glucose again to make sure your level is 70 or above. Repeat these steps until your blood glucose level is 70 or above. Once your blood glucose is stable and if it will be at least an hour before your next meal, have a snack.

If you take diabetes medicines that can cause low blood glucose, always carry food for emergencies. You should also wear a medical identification bracelet or necklace.

Signs of Low Blood Glucose

The signs of low blood glucose include shaking, confusion, extreme hunger, sweating, fatigue, moods swings, experiencing a rapid heart beat or even passing out. You may sweat a lot or get a headache. If your blood glucose drops lower, you could pass out or have a seizure.

Low glucose levels can be caused by:

- type and amount of food - Delaying or skipping a meal, or having a meal with less carbohydrates than you normally have

- more activity than usual - If you increase your level of activity, your blood glucose levels can drop. Whenever you start a new activity, monitor more frequently to watch for glucose changes

- more medication than usual - When you have more medication than normal, an extra dose for example, blood glucose levels can drop

If your blood glucose is low - less than 4mmol/L:

- check your glucose, if you can't test and you have symptoms, begin to treat it

- take 15g of 'fast acting' carbohydrate right away, i.e., 15g glucose tablets or 3 teaspoons of sugar

- wait 15 minutes and recheck your blood glucose, you should be feeling better

- if you are not feeling better, or your glucose level is less than 4 mmol/L, take another 15g of 'fast acting' carbohydrate

- glucose tablets are the preferred method of treating low glucose levels. A few quick sugar remedies are: 1/2 cup orange or apple juice; 1 small box of raisins; 2 teaspoons of honey or sugar; 3 dextrosols or 4 hard candies

- if your next meal is more than 1 hour away, eat a snack of a starch and protein, for example, cheese and 6 crackers; half of a peanut butter or meat sandwich

Some people who take insulin may need a Glucagon Kit available for emergencies. If your blood glucose drops so low that you become unconscious or can't swallow, an injection of *glucagon* may be necessary. Make sure your family, friends, or co-workers are aware of your situation and how to administer *glucagon* in the event you lose consciousness.

If you are taking medication that increases your insulin levels, or if you take insulin injections, you are at risk for low blood glucose.

You can prevent low blood glucose by eating regular meals, taking your diabetes medicines, and checking your blood glucose often. Checking will tell you whether your glucose level is going down. You can then take steps, like drinking fruit juice, to raise your blood glucose.

Keeping a Logbook or Daily Record

Write down each glucose reading and the date and time you took it. When you review your records you can see a pattern of your recent glucose control. Show your blood glucose records to your health care team who will determine whether you need changes in your diabetes medicines or your meal plan. If you don't know what your results mean ask your health care team. You may also want to write down what you ate, how you felt, and whether you exercised.

Things to write down every day in your record book are

- results of your blood glucose checks

- your diabetes medicines: times and amounts taken

- if you ate more or less food than you usually do

- if you were sick

- if you found *ketones* in your blood or urine

- what kind of physical activity you did and for how long

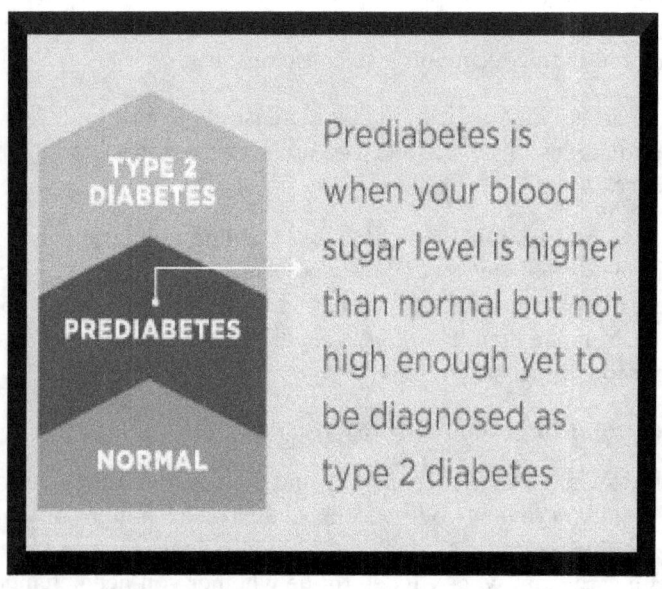

TYPE 2
DIABETES

PREDIABETES

NORMAL

Prediabetes is when your blood sugar level is higher than normal but not high enough yet to be diagnosed as type 2 diabetes

Medications

Treatment of type 2 diabetes begins with lifestyle changes, particularly with diet and exercise. If lifestyle changes don't put blood glucose levels in the target range, medications may be required. People with type 1 diabetes need insulin continuously to survive. Medications for type 2 diabetes include anti-diabetes pills, insulin injections, or a combination of both. A large part of adjusting to life with diabetes involves learning about the many medications that are available to treat the disease and possible complications.

Pills

If your body makes insulin but the insulin doesn't lower your blood glucose enough you may need diabetes pills. Ask your

 health care team when you should take your pills and be sure to tell your doctor if the pills make you feel sick or if you have any other side effects.

Sometimes, people who take diabetes pills may need insulin for a while. If you get sick or have surgery the diabetes pills may no longer work to lower your blood glucose.

You may be able to stop taking diabetes pills if you lose weight. Always check with your doctor before you stop taking your diabetes pills. Losing 10 or 15 pounds can help you reach your target blood glucose levels.

Insulin

You need insulin if your body has stopped making insulin or if it doesn't make enough. Everyone with type 1 diabetes needs insulin and many people with type 2 diabetes do too. Some women with gestational diabetes also need to take insulin.

Your doctor can tell you which of these ways to take insulin is best for you:

- injections - a needle is attached to a syringe that is filled with a dose of insulin. Some people use an *insulin pen* which is a pen-like device with a needle and a cartridge of insulin

- insulin pump - a small device worn on a belt or in a pocket that holds insulin. The pump connects to a small plastic tube and a very small needle which is inserted under the skin and stays in for several days

- insulin jet injector - sends a fine spray of insulin through the skin with high-pressure air instead of a needle

- insulin infuser - a small tube is inserted just beneath the skin and remains in place for several days. Insulin is injected into the end of the tube instead of through the skin

Medications are very effective at treating diabetes and reducing the symptoms and long-term effects of the condition. However, *hypoglycemia* (a blood glucose level that is too low) can occur when taking certain medications for diabetes.

Lifestyle Changes

Lifestyle changes, including healthy eating, weight control, and exercise, can help prevent or delay the onset of type 2 diabetes. Eliminate as much stress from you life as possible. Stress can significantly affect your ability to control the disease. If you are under stress, you may skip meals or forget to take your medicines, which will affect your blood sugar level.

Exercise helps control type 2 diabetes by:

- improves the body's use of insulin

- burns excess body fat, which helps decrease and control weight

- improves muscle strength

- increases bone density and strength

- lowers blood pressure

- reduces stress

Stock the proper tools. Keep plenty of diabetes supplies, such as lancets, testing strips, diabetes medication, syringes, and glucose tablets or juice, on hand. Make sure you have replacement batteries for your glucose meter and an extra pen for recording your blood glucose results. A travel or cosmetics case can keep supplies together, organized, and portable. Consider having two meters, one at home and one at work for easy access.

Purchase appropriate foods to make diabetes care easy for you. If you must buy desserts and other temptations for your family, store them out of sight. Temptation that stares you in the face is hard to resist.

If you find yourself in a slump with your care, enlist the support of family and friends to remind you to keep up with your testing and medication. Bear in mind your testing does not become their responsibility; it is yours.

Devise ways to remind yourself. Leave your meter in an obvious location so you remember to test. Leave yourself notes in conspicuous places. Synchronize the testing and/or medication to coincide with other activities in your daily routine; for example, when the coffee is brewing in the morning, test your blood glucose.

Establish a routine. It sounds so obvious, but if you establish a routine for your care, diabetes management becomes an automatic response, even when you feel stressed or pressured by other events in your life.

Don't let diabetes care keep you from doing something you really want to do. With frequent testing and a good understanding of your diabetes care, you can participate in most activities you enjoy.

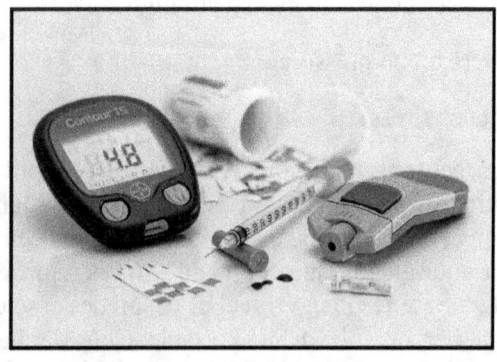

Diabetes Diet

A healthy diet is key to controlling blood sugar levels and preventing diabetes complications.

a) If the patient is obese and has had difficulty losing weight on their own, talk to a health care professional. He or she can recommend a dietitian or a weight modification program to help the patient reach a goal.

b) Eat a consistent, well-balanced diet that is high in fiber, low in saturated fat, and low in concentrated sweets.

c) A consistent diet that includes roughly the same number of calories at about the same times of day helps the health care professional prescribe the correct dose of medication or insulin.

d) A healthy diet also helps to keep blood sugar at a relatively even level and avoids excessively low or high blood sugar levels, which can be dangerous and even life-threatening.

Diet Tips

Your diet is very important for preventing, treating, and controlling type 2 diabetes. It is possible to avoid diabetes by maintaining healthy eating habits. Foods that are low in fat and free of partially hydrogenated fat can help people avoid diabetes. Vegetable oils, nuts, and seeds are ideal replacements for meat and dairy products that are high in fat. It is advisable to eat lean meats when possible.

After a diabetes diagnosis, people will need to be stricter with their diets. Patients with diabetes must avoid smoking and must limit and regulate how much sugar they consume. A controlled diet, when coupled with exercise, can keep diabetes and blood sugar under control.

You may need to work with a doctor to adjust your diet if you are taking part in an exercise or fitness program. Physical activity is important, especially if you have diabetes; however, working out can change how your body metabolizes energy.

You will need to test your glucose levels frequently to make sure that your levels remain within a desirable range. You may need to check your blood sugar before meals, after meals, before you exercise, and after you exercise.

You can take good care of yourself and your diabetes by learning:

- what to eat

- how much to eat

- when to eat

Making wise food choices can help you:

- feel good every day

- lose weight if you need to

- lower your risk for heart disease, stroke, and other problems caused by diabetes

Healthful eating helps keep your blood glucose, also called blood sugar, in your target range. Physical activity and, if needed, diabetes medicines also help. The diabetes target range is the blood glucose level suggested by diabetes experts for good health. You can help prevent health problems by keeping your blood glucose levels on target.

Choose high-fiber, slow-release carbs

Carbohydrates have a big impact on your blood sugar levels -
more so than fats and proteins - but you don't have to avoid
them. You just need to be smart about what types of carbs you
eat.

In general, it's best to limit highly refined carbohydrates like
white bread, pasta, and rice, as well as soda, candy, and snack
foods. Focus instead on high-fiber complex carbohydrates - also
known as slow-release carbs. Slow-release carbs help keep blood
sugar levels even because they are digested more slowly, thus
preventing your body from producing too much insulin. They
also provide lasting energy and help you stay full longer.

What is also important is to eat enough fat. If you try to cut back
on carbs and fat, you will end up ravenously hungry and feel
miserable.

What foods are slow-release?

Several tools have been designed to help answer this question.
The glycemic index (GI) tells you how quickly a food turns into
sugar in your system. Glycemic load, a newer term, looks at both
the glycemic index and the amount of carbohydrate in a food,
giving you a more accurate idea of how a food may affect your
blood sugar level. High GI foods spike your blood sugar rapidly,
while low GI foods have the least effect.

You can find glycemic index and glycemic load tables online,
but you don't have to rely on food charts in order to make smart
choices. Australian chef Michael Moore has come up with an
easier way to regulate the carbs you eat. He classifies foods into
three broad categories: fire, water, and coal. The harder your
body needs to work to break food down, the better.

Fire foods have a high GI, and are low in fiber and protein. They
include "white foods" (white rice, white pasta, white bread,
potatoes, most baked goods), sweets, chips, and many processed
foods. They should be limited in your diet.

Water foods are free foods - meaning you can eat as many as you
like. They include all vegetables and most types of fruit (fruit

juice, dried fruit, and canned fruit packed in syrup spike blood sugar quickly and are not considered water foods).

Coal foods have a low GI and are high in fiber and protein. They include nuts and seeds, lean meats, seafood, whole grains, and beans. They also include "white food" replacements such as brown rice, whole-wheat bread, and whole-wheat pasta.

8 principles of low-glycemic eating

1. Eat a lot of non-starchy vegetables, beans, and fruits such as apples, pears, peaches, and berries. Even tropical fruits like bananas, mangoes, and papayas tend to have a lower glycemic index than typical desserts.

2. Eat grains in the least-processed state possible: "unbroken," such as whole-kernel bread, brown rice, and whole barley, millet, and wheat berries; or traditionally processed, such as stone-ground bread, steel-cut oats, and natural granola or muesli breakfast cereals.

3. Limit white potatoes and refined grain products such as white breads and white pasta to small side dishes.

4. Limit concentrated sweets - including high-calorie foods with a low glycemic index, such as ice cream - to occasional treats. Reduce fruit juice to no more than one cup a day. Completely eliminate sugar-sweetened drinks.

5. Eat a healthful type of protein at most meals, such as beans, fish, or skinless chicken.

6. Choose foods with healthful fats, such as olive oil, nuts (almonds, walnuts, pecans), and avocados. Limit saturated fats from dairy and other animal products. Completely eliminate partially hydrogenated fats (trans fats), which are in fast food and many packaged foods.

7. Have three meals and one or two snacks each day, and don't skip breakfast.

8. Eat slowly and stop when full.

Adapted from Ending the Food Fight, by David Ludwig with Suzanne Rostler (Houghton Mifflin, 2008).

Be smart about sweets

Eating for diabetes doesn't mean eliminating sugar. If you have diabetes, you can still enjoy a small serving of your favourite dessert now and then. The key is moderation.

But maybe you have a sweet tooth and the thought of cutting back on sweets sounds almost as bad as cutting them out altogether. The good news is that cravings do go away and preferences change. As your eating habits become healthier, foods that you used to love may seem too rich or too sweet, and you may find yourself craving healthier options.

How to include sweets in a diabetes-friendly diet

a) Hold the bread (or rice or pasta) if you want dessert. Eating sweets at a meal adds extra carbohydrates. Because of this it is best to cut back on the other carb-containing foods at the same meal.

b) Add some healthy fat to your dessert. It may seem counter-intuitive to pass over the low-fat or fat-free desserts in favour of their higher-fat counterparts. But fat slows down the digestive process, meaning blood sugar levels don't spike as quickly. That doesn't mean, however, that you should reach for the donuts. Think healthy fats, such as peanut butter, ricotta cheese, yogurt, or some nuts.

c) Eat sweets with a meal, rather than as a stand-alone snack. When eaten on their own, sweets and desserts cause your blood sugar to spike. But if you eat them along with other healthy foods as part of your meal, your blood sugar won't rise as rapidly.

d) When you eat dessert, truly savour each bite. How many times have you mindlessly eaten your way through a bag of cookies or a huge piece of cake. Can you really say that you enjoyed each bite? Make your indulgence count by eating slowly and paying attention to the flavours and textures. You'll enjoy it more, plus you're less likely to overeat.

Tricks for cutting down on sugar

1. Reduce how much soda and juice you drink. If you miss your carbonation kick, try sparkling water either plain or with a little juice mixed in.

2. Reduce the amount of sugar in recipes by ¼ to ⅓. If a recipe calls for 1 cup of sugar, for example, use ⅔ or ¾ cup instead. You can also boost sweetness with cinnamon, nutmeg, or vanilla extract.

3. Find healthy ways to satisfy your sweet tooth. Instead of ice cream, blend up frozen bananas for a creamy, frozen treat. Or enjoy a small chunk of dark chocolate, rather than your usual milk chocolate bar.

4. Start with half of the dessert you normally eat, and replace the other half with fruit.

Proceed with caution when it comes to alcohol

It's easy to underestimate the amount of calories and carbs in alcoholic drinks, including beer and wine. Cocktails mixed with soda and juice can be loaded with sugar. If you're going to drink, do so in moderation (no more than 1 drink per day for women; 2 for men), choose calorie-free drink mixers, and drink only with food. If you're diabetic, always monitor your blood glucose, as alcohol can interfere with diabetes medication and insulin. Excessive alcohol use is a known risk factor for type 2 diabetes. Alcohol consumption can cause low or high blood sugar levels, nerve pain (neuritis), and an increase in triglycerides.

Choose fats wisely

Fats can be either helpful or harmful in your diet. People with diabetes are at higher risk for heart disease, so it is even more important to be smart about fats. Some fats are unhealthy and others have enormous health benefits. But all fats are high in calories, so you should always watch your portion sizes.

- **Unhealthy fats** - The two most damaging fats are saturated fats and trans fats. Saturated fats are found mainly in animal products such as red meat, whole milk dairy products, and eggs. Trans fats, also called partially hydrogenated oils, are created by adding hydrogen to liquid vegetable oils to make them more solid and less likely to spoil - which is very good for food manufacturers, and very bad for you.

- **Healthy fats** - The best fats are unsaturated fats, which come from plant and fish sources and are liquid at room temperature. Primary sources include olive oil, canola oil, nuts, and avocados. Also focus on omega-3 fatty acids, which fight inflammation and support brain and heart health. Good sources include salmon, tuna, and flax seeds.

Ways to reduce unhealthy fats and add healthy fats

1. Cook with olive oil instead of butter or vegetable oil.

2. Trim any visible fat off of meat before cooking and remove the skin before cooking chicken and turkey.

3. Instead of chips or crackers, try snacking on nuts or seeds. Add them to your morning cereal or have a little handful for a filling snack. Nut butters are also very satisfying and full of healthy fats.

4. Instead of frying, choose to grill, broil, bake, or stir-fry.

5. Serve fish 2 or 3 times week instead of red meat.

6. Add avocado to your sandwiches instead of cheese. This will keep the creamy texture, but improve the health factor.

7. When baking, use canola oil or applesauce instead of shortening or butter.

8. Rather than using heavy cream, make your soups creamy by adding low-fat milk thickened with flour, pureed potatoes, or reduced-fat sour cream.

Try Something Different

Filling your grocery cart with the same broccoli, pasta, and chicken week after week can get boring very quickly. Try something different with these nutritious foods:

Soynuts

They have 40 per cent fewer calories than peanuts, but the same satisfying crunch and heart health benefits. Look for them in the bulk food section or snack aisle. They are a nutritious snack, nut-free and school safe and can be pureed into soynut butter. Just one quarter cup (50 mL) has an impressive 5 grams of fibre and 10 grams of protein.

Kohlrabi

This bulbous vegetable with a leafy green top has a mild flavour reminiscent of broccoli, and it's high in vitamin C. Peel the hard outer layer, shred it raw into a salad; cube and roast with other vegetables; stir-fry leaves with garlic and olive oil.

Kefir

This tart and tangy fermented dairy beverage is usually alongside milk or near yogurt. Kefir is filled with healthy probiotics and is rich in calcium. Choose one made from skim or 2% milk, without added sugar. Pour on cereal, muesli or granola, or drink as is.

Rye crackers

Found in the deli aisle or the top shelf in the cracker aisle, these may be called crispbread or flatbread. They have two simple ingredients: whole grain rye flour and salt (although low in sodium). Use them to replace crackers made with refined white flour.

Frozen dark leafy greens

If fresh kale and spinach end up wilting in your fridge, buy frozen instead. Their vitamins and minerals are locked in by quick freezing within hours of picking. Add a handful of greens to soup, pasta, eggs, wraps and rice dishes, or stir-fry and serve as a side dish.

Greek yogurt

Find it beside other yogurts, and choose one that's lowest in sugar (less than 10 g per 175 mL serving). Thick and creamy, and with double the protein of traditional yogurt, Greek yogurt is a perfect replacement for sour cream or an ideal any time snack. Use it as a base for dips or in desserts. Greek yogurt, when compared with regular yogurt, has twice the protein.

Calamari

If looking for a kid-friendly, inexpensive, nutritious protein option that you can prepare in just two minutes consider a bag of frozen squid rings or calamari. Their fun shape and mild flavour make them perfect for picky eaters. Dress with olive oil, lemon juice and Italian herbs, and grill or sauté for two minutes.

Millet

Used as a whole grain, millet is actually a seed from tall grass grown primarily in Asia and Africa. Look for puffed millet in the cereal aisle, or millet grain in the bulk section. The grain cooks to a mashed potato-like consistency, and makes a high fibre, iron-rich substitute for rice, pasta and potatoes. Blend cooked millet with your favourite savoury herbs and spices, or add cinnamon and raisins for breakfast.

Dried figs

If you're bored of raisins try this year-round staple as your go-to dried fruit. Find packaged figs near fresh fruit or in the bulk aisle. They are rich in fibre, calcium, iron and potassium, figs also satisfy a sweet tooth. Skip the cookies and enjoy two figs instead. Add chopped figs to quinoa, salads or yogurt or stuff them with goat cheese for yummy appetizers.

Lentils

Lentils can be found dried or canned (look for "no added salt" if buying canned). They are rich in fibre and iron, and dried lentils cook quickly and require no soaking. Red lentils are the quickest to cook and are perfect for soup or millet burgers. Larger green lentils are great in bean salads, pilafs and stews. Add pureed lentils to lasagna, dips and muffins.

Eat all you like

- **Meat**: Any type, including beef, pork, game meat, chicken, etc. Feel free to eat the fat on the meat as well as the skin on the chicken. If possible try to choose organic or grass fed meat.

- **Fish and shellfish**: All kinds: Fatty fish such as salmon, mackerel or herring are great. Avoid breading.

- **Eggs**: All kinds: Boiled, fried, omelettes, etc. Preferably organic eggs.

- **Natural fat, high-fat sauces:** Using butter and cream for cooking can make your food taste better and make you feel more satiated. Try a Béarnaise or Hollandaise sauce, check the ingredients or make it yourself. Coconut oil and olive oil are also good options.

- **Vegetables that grow above ground**: All kinds of cabbage, such as cauliflower, broccoli, cabbage and Brussels sprouts. Asparagus, zucchini, eggplant, olives, spinach, mushrooms, cucumber, lettuce, avocado, onions, peppers, tomatoes etc.

- **Dairy products**: Always select full-fat options like real butter, cream (40% fat), sour cream, Greek/Turkish yogurt and high-fat cheeses. Be careful with regular milk and skim milk as they contain a lot of milk sugar. Avoid flavored, sugary and low-fat products.

- **Nuts**: Great for a TV treat instead of candy (ideally in moderation).

- **Berries**: Okay in moderation, if you are not a super strict or sensitive. Great with whipped cream.

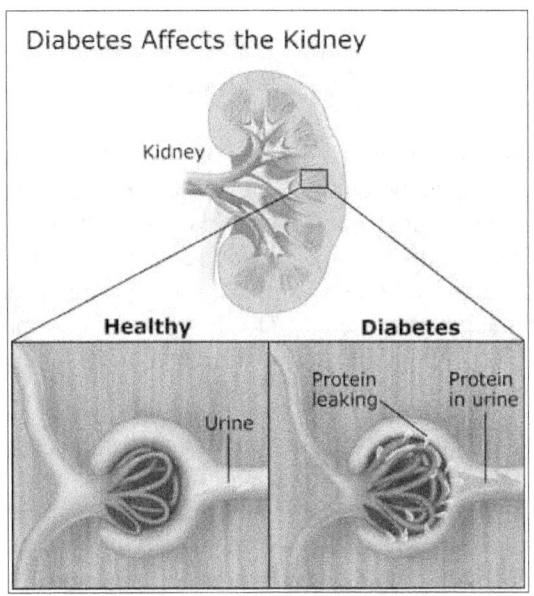

Snacking

Snacking is a part of our lives that is meant to tide us over, not replace a meal, and we shouldn't have to give it up because we are changing our lifestyle. Deprivation will probably result in over indulgence some time in the future, so to prevent this simply change what you snack on. Choosing healthy snacks not only keep hunger pangs at bay, and conquer the mid-morning and mid-afternoon fatigue, but will keep you feeling energized throughout the day.

Planning your snacks will avoid making unhealthy choices that may be high in salt, fat, or sugar. Not only will potato chips, cookies, doughnuts, and candy bars actually sap your energy, they will pile on the calories. Snacking on half a whole-grain bagel spread with low-fat cheese, or a handful of nuts with an apple, will boost your energy and leave you feeling satisfied longer.

When it comes to successful weight loss, research shows that the two most helpful strategies involve following a regular eating schedule and recording what you eat.

Stock up your pantry and fridge with quick and easy choices, such as:

- fresh fruit

- sliced vegetables

- plain popcorn

- unsalted nuts

- dried fruit

- trail mix

- single servings of low-fat yogurt or cottage cheese

At work keep a snacking survival kit at your desk or in your locker, or in your purse or briefcase, filled with:

- whole grain crackers

- peanut butter

- canned fruit

- nuts and seeds

- dried fruit

- unsalted nuts

- low-fat cereal bars

- trail mix

Outdoor summer activities, such as amusement parks, long drives in the country, bike riding, or a long hike, will make you hungry. We can't get through summer without an ice-cream cone, or two, or cups of special coffee blends, but even these treats can be kept to a minimum. Packing your own snacks will spare both your wallet and your waistline.

Choose snacks that have protein, fibre, and good carbs for energy.

Fresh fruits have high water content that will keep your hydrated, such as:

- watermelon

- oranges

- strawberries

- honeydew melon

- grapes

- peaches

- apricots

Sliced vegetable sticks in an enticing array of colours, or loose bunches, such as:

- carrots

- green or yellow beans

- celery

- cucumbers

- asparagus

- sweet peppers

- broccoli

- cauliflower

Trail Mix is a must-have snack. Remember there are plenty of calories in fruit and nuts so keep your blend higher in cereal and portions to half a cup. Make your own Trail Mix that is filling and nutritious with:

- nuts

- seeds

- dried fruit

- whole grain cereal

- air-popped corn

Pack some non-perishable proteins such as:

- nut and seed butters (peanut, almond, cashew, sunflower, soy)

- mini cans of tuna

- cheese or hummus (if you have an ice pack)

Include fibre-rich grains, such as:

- whole grain rye crackers

- corn tortillas

- brown rice cakes

- whole grain breads, bagels, or muffins

Making healthy choices at convenience stores, coffee shops, or fast food outlets, can be a challenge but many shops are stocking better snacks, such as:

- energy bars with whole ingredients: soy, oats, nuts and dried fruit

- yogurt blended with fruit and cereal

- nuts and seeds (always a smart choice as long as they aren't covered in salt or chocolate)

- milk

Late Night Snacking

Usually eating dinner 3-4 hours before bedtime and having a small snack 1-2 hours before going to sleep will give your body a chance to digest foods and allow your stomach to settle so you can get a good night's rest. Eating after dinner is not always a bad thing as long as your food choices are not high in calories and fat. Here are a few tips to curb late night snacking:

- know when to stop – our body requires the least amount of energy at night. Any extra calories not used for energy will be stored as fat.

- don't eat from the box or bag – measure out your portion so you know how much you're eating.

- emotional eating – whether it's stress, TV commercials, boredom, find another way to help you cope such as reading a book, phoning a friend, or going for a walk

- satisfying a sweet tooth – choose oranges or berries, or combine fresh fruit or high-fibre cereal with low-fat yogurt.

Cravings

If you crave ice cream or french fries after a bad day at work or a fight with your spouse, you are not alone. There's a reason your brain wants sweet and high-fat foods when you're feeling tense.

The problem is that chronic stress - and too many french fries - can contribute to weight gain and the health problems that accompany it. Can you have your cake and eat it too? Yes you can, if you choose smaller portions of better-for-you comfort foods that are delicious and nutritious.

People who keep a food diary lose twice as much weight as those who don't.

Stress eating

The relationship between high stress lifestyles and growing waistlines is not a coincidence. Researchers are slowly unravelling how brain chemistry drives our food choices, and why stress may lead you to eat. While the science is far from complete, the work to date is fascinating.

Hormones such as leptin, ghrelin and cortisol are part of the complex equation that regulates appetite, sleep, stress and weight. A balanced diet, paired with physical activity and adequate sleep, can help ensure proper levels of these hormones, and help keep your weight in check.

When the hormones are out of balance, and when sleep and chronic stress come into play, you may crave more sweet and fatty foods.

Comfort foods

In times of stress, you may turn to creamy pasta casserole, or you may prefer sweet snacks like chocolate and ice cream. Regardless of your choice, comfort foods that contain sugar, fat, or both, are reported to help ease tension and produce mild feelings of happiness.

Several researchers have proposed that high-fat food (think macaroni and cheese, ice cream, french fries) may trigger the brain's "pleasure pathway." And sugar helps the body produce serotonin, a neurotransmitter that promotes happiness and a sense of well-being.

So, it's a catch-22. Comfort foods really do help ease stress and make you feel good, but they also contribute to obesity. Is there a way to get the stress-busting benefits without the calories? Yes! Even small servings of sweet or fatty foods – like a half-cup of ice cream or a Halloween-sized chocolate bar – can alter a negative mood.

Eat well, feel great

The effect on your mood is the same whether your sugar comes from fruit or candy, so opt for watermelon, berries or peaches instead of gummy bears. When choosing fatty foods, try foods made with oil instead of butter, lard or shortening, and keep the portions small.

Here are some great recipes to ease stress while keeping your diet in check:

If you like creamy: Try an almond rice pudding. It provides sweetness from dates instead of sugar, and has a creamy mouth feel with fewer calories than ice cream. Bonus: it's made with whole grains!

If you like comforting casseroles: Try a meaty Shepherd's pie with garlic mash, which includes classic, comforting potatoes made extra creamy by being mashed with beans.

If you crave chocolate: Make muffins with canola oil instead of butter. Bonus: a portion-controlled muffin freeze well - just take one from the freezer when a comfort food craving hits.

Desserts

Dessert has a place in a nutritious diet, as long as you observe the rules of moderation. Dessert can be as simple as a bowl of grapes or a crunchy apple. However, to most people, dessert is anything decadent that's made with sugar, such as ice cream, cookies, pie or cake.

Fruit is something that can naturally be included after every meal. Even a square or two of good quality dark chocolate can be part of a healthy diet most days and there are very tasty sugar free chocolate brands available. But if your idea of dessert is calorie-rich premium ice cream or lemon meringue pie, you need to be mindful about your indulgence.

There are four things to consider if you want to make dessert a healthy part of your lifestyle:

1. How often?

Eating high-calorie, sweet and fatty desserts after every meal is a quick route to weight gain and associated problems such as high blood sugar and hypertension. High-calorie desserts should be a trat that you enjoy occasionally, not daily.

2. How much?

There's a big difference between ending your meal with two small cookies (100 calories) or with a caramel fudge marshmallow explosion cake (800 calories). Yes, dessert tastes good, but eating more of it won't make it taste better. Stick with a treat in the 100-200 calorie range; that will keep you satisfied but not feeling gluttonous.

3. What counts?

Be honest with yourself about which foods are dessert items so you can accurately monitor your intake. A donut or Danish at your morning coffee break, a calorie-laden frozen coffee drink or a fruit smoothie counts as dessert too!

4. What's inside?

Whole foods like nuts, fruit and oats are the foundations of healthy desserts, as long as they don't come wrapped in too much butter and sugar. For better-for-you desserts:

- o   Use fruit as a main ingredient

- o   Bake with whole grain oat, rice, barley or wheat flour

- o   Use antioxidant-rich cocoa or dark chocolate instead of milk chocolate

- o   Bake with oil instead of butter, shortening or lard

- o   Replace up to half the fat with applesauce or jarred prunes.

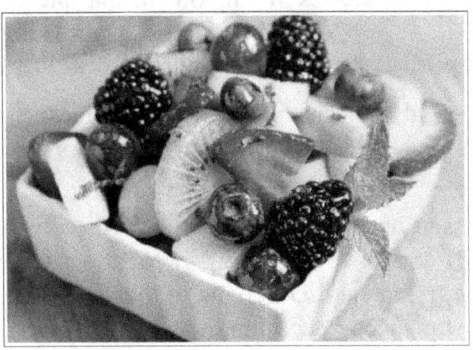

Here are some lightened-up ways to enjoy the desserts you crave, but with fewer calories and less fat.

If you enjoy...	Try this instead...
Premium ice cream (290 calories per ½ cup)	Frozen yogurt (140 calories per ½ cup)
Apple pie (300 calories per 125 g slice)	Apple crisp (200 calories per 125 g serving)
Fudgy brownies (243 calories per brownie)	Reduced-fat Double chocolate brownies* (111 calories per brownie)
Pannacotta with heavy cream (418 calories per serving)	Strawberry pomegranate pannacotta * (87 calories per serving)
Pumpkin pie (316 calories per slice)	Pumpkin banana spiced custard * (111 calories per serving)
Berry sundae (341 calories per serving)	Berries with a tablespoon of whipped cream (100 calories per serving)

Enjoying dessert once in a while is a perfectly sensible indulgence. If you crave something sweet after dinner, have fruit most often or try a healthier version of the dessert you love. Save rich desserts for special occasions.

Dessert Recipes

* Strawberry and pomegranate pannacotta

Makes 6 servings

Ingredients

> 1 cup (250 mL) 2% milk
> ½ cup (125 mL) 1% buttermilk
> ½ cup (125 mL) fresh pomegranate juice
> ¼ cup (50 mL) sugar-free, seedless strawberry jam
> 1 envelope plain gelatin (enough to set 2 cups/500 mL)
> 3 cups (750 mL) fresh strawberries, sliced
> Fresh pomegranate seeds (optional)

Directions:

1. In a medium bowl, combine milk, buttermilk, juice and jam.

2. Make gelatin according to package instructions. Whisk into the milk mixture.

3. Pour into six ramekins and let set in the fridge for at least 3 hours or overnight.

4. To remove the pannacotta from the ramekins, place the ramekin into very hot water for 1 minute. Run a sharp knife along the inside edge of the ramekin and invert onto the individual serving plate.

5. Garnish with fresh strawberries and pomegranate seeds (if using).

Oatmeal Cranberry Cookies

Ingredients

> 1 1/2 cups (375 mL) large flake oats
> 1 cup (250 mL) wheat bran
> ¾ cup (175 mL) whole-wheat flour
> ½ tsp (2 mL) baking soda
> ½ tsp (2 mL) ground cinnamon
> 2/3 cup (150 mL) packed brown sugar
> 1/4 cup (50 mL) non-hydrogenated soft margarine
> 1/4 cup (50 mL) orange juice
> 2 egg whites
> 2 tsp (10 mL) vanilla
> 1/2 tsp (2 mL) grated orange rind
> ½ cup (125 mL) chopped dried cranberries or currants

Directions:

1. In a bowl, whisk together oats, bran, flour, baking soda and cinnamon; set aside.

2. In another large bowl, beat sugar, margarine, egg whites, orange juice, vanilla and orange rind until smooth. Add oat mixture to bowl and stir until combined. Add cranberries and stir to combine.

3. Drop dough by tablespoonfuls (15 mL) on parchment paper lined baking sheet and flatten slightly.

4. Bake in 375 F (190 C) oven for about 15 minutes or until firm and golden. Repeat with remaining dough. Let cool on rack.

Storage: Keep in airtight container for up to 3 days or freeze for up to 1 month.

Double chocolate brownies

Makes 16 brownies

These rich-tasting brownies are amazingly low in calories.

Ingredients

> 150 mL (2⁄3 cup) all-purpose flour
> 125 mL (1⁄2 cup) granulated sugar
> 75 mL (1⁄3 cup) unsweetened cocoa powder
> 5 mL (1 tsp) baking powder
> 1 mL (1⁄4 tsp) or less salt
> 5 mL (1 tsp) pure vanilla extract
> 5 mL (1 tsp) instant coffee granules
> 50 mL (1⁄4 cup) soft margarine
> 2 eggs
> 125 mL (1⁄2 cup) unsweetened applesauce
> 125 mL (1⁄2 cup) chocolate chips

Directions:

1. In bowl, stir together flour, sugar, cocoa, baking powder and salt.

2. Mix vanilla and coffee to dissolve coffee.

3. In mixing bowl, beat margarine, eggs and vanilla mixture for 1 minute.

4. Add applesauce and beat just until blended.

5. Fold in flour mixture and chocolate chips just until blended.

6. Spread evenly in greased 8-inch (2 L) square pan. Bake in 350°F (180°C) oven for about 12 minutes until outside edges are firm. Cool on rack.

Store in covered container in refrigerator for up to 1 week.

Chocolate Walnut Brownies

Ingredients

   1 can (19 oz/540 mL) white kidney beans, drained and
   rinsed
   2/3 cup (150 mL) packed brown sugar
   ½ cup (125 mL) skim milk
   2 egg whites
   ¼ cup (50 mL) soft non-hydrogenated margarine, melted
   1 tbsp (15 mL) vanilla
   ½ cup (125 mL) whole-wheat flour
   ½ cup (125 mL) unsweetened cocoa powder
   1/3 cup (75 mL) wheat germ
   1 tsp (5 mL) baking powder
   1/3 cup (75 mL) chopped toasted walnuts

Directions:

1. In food processor, puree beans until coarse. Add in
    sugar, milk, egg whites, margarine and vanilla and puree
    until smooth, scraping down sides a few times.

2. In a large bowl whisk together flour, cocoa, wheat germ
    and baking powder. Pour bean mixture over flour
    mixture. Stir in walnuts to combine. Scrape batter into
    parchment paper lined 8-inch (1.5 L) square baking pan,
    smoothing top.

3. Bake in 350F (180 C) oven for about 22 minutes or until
    cake tester inserted comes out clean. Let cool on rack.

* Pumpkin banana spiced custard

Makes 6 servings

Ingredients

> 1 egg
> 2 egg whites
> 1 cup (250 ml) canned pure pumpkin
> 1/3 cup (75 mL) mashed banana (1 medium)
> 1 cup (250 mL) evaporated skim milk
> ¼ cup (50 mL) packed brown sugar
> ½ tsp (2 ml) ground cinnamon
> ¼ tsp (1 mL) ground ginger
> 1/8 tsp (0.5 mL) allspice
> 6 walnut halves

Directions:

1. Preheat oven to 325° F (160° C).

2. Place 6 1 cup (250 mL) ramekins in a glass 13 x 9 inch (3.5 L) baking dish.

3. In a large bowl, combine all the ingredients except the walnut halves. Pour custard into ramekins. Pour boiling water around the ramekins in the baking dish to a depth of 1 inch (2.5 cm). Place 1 walnut half in the centre of each custard.

4. Bake for 40 minutes. Remove from the oven and serve warm.

Weight Loss

If you're overweight, you may be encouraged to note that you only have to lose 7% of your body weight to cut your risk of diabetes in half. And you don't have to obsessively count calories or starve yourself to do it.

When it comes to successful weight loss, research shows that the two most helpful strategies involve following a regular eating schedule and recording what you eat.

Eat at regularly set times

Your body is better able to regulate blood sugar levels - and your weight - when you maintain a regular meal schedule. Aim for moderate and consistent portion sizes for each meal or snack.

Don't skip breakfast. Start your day off with a good breakfast. Eating breakfast every day will help you have energy as well as steady blood sugar levels.

Eat regular small meals - up to 6 per day. People tend to eat larger portions when they are overly hungry, so eating regularly will help you keep your portions in check.

Keep calorie intake the same. Regulating the amount of calories you eat on a day-to-day basis has an impact on the regularity of your blood sugar levels. Try to eat roughly the same amount of calories every day, rather than overeating one day or at one meal, and then skimping on the next.

Keep a food diary

Research shows that people who keep a food diary are more likely to lose weight and keep it off. In fact, a recent study found that people who kept a food diary lost twice as much weight as those who didn't.

Why does writing down what you eat and drink help you drop pounds? For one, it helps you identify problem areas - such as your afternoon snack or your morning latte - where you're getting a lot more calories than you realized. It also increases your awareness of what, why, and how much you're eating, which helps you cut back on mindless snacking and emotional eating.

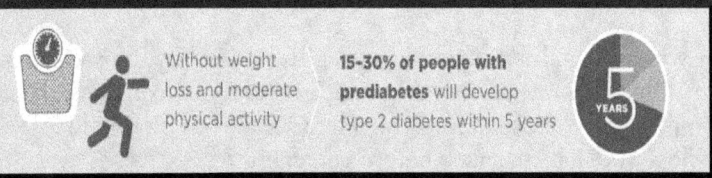

Without weight loss and moderate physical activity **15-30% of people with prediabetes** will develop type 2 diabetes within 5 years

Exercise

Before you begin exercising, talk with your doctor. Your doctor may check your heart and your feet to be sure you have no special problems. If you have high blood pressure or eye problems, some exercises like weightlifting may not be safe. Your health care team can help you find safe exercises.

When it comes to preventing, controlling, or reversing diabetes, you can't afford to overlook exercise. Exercise can help your weight loss efforts, and is especially important in maintaining weight loss. There is also evidence that regular exercise can improve your insulin sensitivity even if you don't lose weight.

You don't have to become a gym rat or adopt a gruelling fitness regimen. One of the easiest ways is to start walking for 30 minutes five or more times a week. You can also try swimming, biking, or any other moderate-intensity activities - meaning you work up a light sweat and start to breathe harder. Even house and yard work counts.

Try to be active almost every day for a total of about 30 minutes. If you haven't been very active lately, begin slowly. Start with 5 to 10 minutes, and then add more time. Or exercise for 10 minutes, three times a day.

If you use insulin or take diabetes pills that help your body make insulin, you may need to eat a snack before you exercise. Check your blood glucose before you exercise. If your blood glucose is below 100, have a snack before you exercise.

When you exercise, carry glucose tablets or a **carbohydrate** snack with you in case you have low blood glucose. Wear or carry an identification tag or card that says you have diabetes.

Physical Activity Plan

What you eat and when also depend on how much you exercise. Physical activity is an important part of staying healthy and controlling your blood glucose. Keep these points in mind:

1. Talk with your doctor about what types of exercise are safe for you.

2. Make sure your shoes fit well and your socks stay clean and dry. Check your feet for redness or sores after exercising. Call your doctor if you have sores that do not heal.

3. Warm up and stretch for 5 to 10 minutes before you exercise. Then cool down for several minutes after you exercise. For example, walk slowly at first, stretch, and then walk faster. Finish up by walking slowly again.

4. Ask your doctor whether you should exercise if your blood glucose level is high.

5. Ask your doctor whether you should have a snack before you exercise.

6. Know the signs of low blood glucose, also called hypoglycemia. Always carry food or glucose tablets to treat low blood glucose.

7. Always wear your medical identification or other ID.

8. Find an exercise buddy. Many people find they are more likely to do something active if a friend joins them. Regular exercise, in any form, can help reduce the risk of developing diabetes. Activity can also reduce the risk of developing complications of diabetes such as heart disease, stroke, kidney failure, blindness, and leg ulcers.

9. As little as 20 minutes of walking three times a week has a proven beneficial effect. Any exercise is beneficial; no

matter how easy or how long, some exercise is better than no exercise.

10. If the patient has complications of diabetes (such as eye, kidney, or nerve problems), they may be limited both in type of exercise, and amount of exercise they can safely do without worsening their condition. Consult with your health care professional before starting any exercise program.

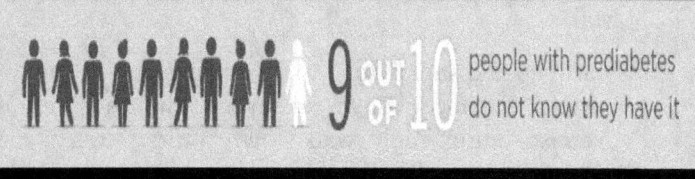

9 OUT OF 10 people with prediabetes do not know they have it

Smoking

If the patient has diabetes, and smokes cigarettes or use any other form of tobacco, they are raising the risks markedly for nearly all of the complications of diabetes. Smoking damages blood vessels and contributes to heart disease, stroke, and poor circulation in the limbs. If a person needs help to quit tobacco use, talk to a health care professional.

Self-monitored blood glucose: Check blood sugar levels frequently, at least before meals and at bedtime, then record the results in a logbook.

This log should also include insulin or oral medication doses and times, when and what the patient ate, when and for how long they exercised, and any significant events of the day such as high or low blood sugar levels and how they treated the problem.

Better equipment now available makes testing blood sugar levels less painful and less complicated than ever. A daily blood sugar diary is invaluable to the health care professional in evaluating how the patient is responding to medications, diet, and exercise in the treatment of diabetes.

Natural/Herbal Remedies

Although up to 30% of people with diabetes use herbal products to help control blood sugar, there are not enough good quality studies to show that these treatments are safe and effective.

Alfalfa

Rich in vitamins, minerals and other nutrients, Alfalfa makes an amazing herbal remedy to lower blood sugar levels.

- Take one teaspoon of Alfalfa seeds and sprinkle them on every meal you eat.

- Alfalfa capsules can also be taken following the directions on the package.

Apple Cider Vinegar

The nutritional components of Apple Cider Vinegar help control the rise in blood sugar levels when you eat a meal.

- Take 2 tablespoons of apple cider vinegar and add a pinch of salt to it.

- Mix it in a glass of water.

- Drink this before every large meal.

Basil

Basil leaves have been shown to lower blood sugar levels. Cactus juice from pods, sometimes found in produce markets or grown in arid climates, is also helpful.

Bilberry

The leaves of the bilberry plant are known to lower blood sugar levels, but don't try to self-medicate your diabetes -- contact a nutritionally trained health care provider before changing your regimen. The berries of this wild perennial help people with diabetes avoid some of the typical complications that are usually related to diminished blood circulation. They have compounds in them that improve circulation and help keep blood cells from clumping together. Their flavonoids keep tiny blood capillaries strong so blood can continue to circulate to all parts of the body.

Bitter Gourd

It is also known as Bitter Gourd Momordica-charantia. After many successful scientific studies, it has been demonstrated very effective to diabetics.

It has been shown to have high content in insulin, which your body starves when you're diabetic. In this way, it helps lowering your sugar blood levels.

Bitter Melon

Take bitter melon juice 2 times a day on empty stomach. Or cook it as a vegetable when preparing your daily dishes or salads.

Cayenne

Cayenne can increase your metabolism and help lose weight, however, if you aren't used to cayenne, start with small proportions and slowly increase the amount over time.

Chromium

Chromium Picolate, the active form of Chromium in our body, plays a crucial role as a natural remedy for diabetes. Chromium affects the number of receptors for insulin, in this way it helps insulin work. Additionally, it can reduce cholesterol and prevent the onset of severe diabetes complications.

Cinnamon

Research has shown that small doses of Cinnamon can be beneficial in treating Type 2 Diabetes, since it can reduce blood sugar levels while simultaneously increasing the body's natural production of insulin.

- Take half a teaspoon of Cinnamon powder each morning.

- Repeat this for 40 days.

Cinnamon powder can be consumed in a number of ways:

- Sprinkle cinnamon into your coffee.

- Add a cinnamon stick to your favorite herbal tea.

- Mix cinnamon powder into unsweetened applesauce.

- Add cinnamon powder to your cereal or oatmeal.

NOTE: If you are taking medication to control blood sugar levels, any regular consumption of cinnamon should only be taken after consulting with your doctor.

Fenugreek

Fenugreek seeds, when dried, can be used in food preparation. The seeds contain an amino acid that may stimulate the secretion of insulin through the pancreas. It also reduces insulin resistance and as a result, blood sugar levels ay be lower. Another component of fenugreek is it contains alkaloids such as gentianine, trigonelline, and carpaine.

Fiber

Eating a diet rich in fiber helps the body absorb sugars slowly, which in turn keeps blood sugar levels on a more even keel. Most of the vegetables and fruits in your garden are rich in fiber. The soluble type of fiber, the one that does the best job of stabilizing blood sugar levels, is abundant in apples, apricots, beets, berries, carrots, citrus fruits, parsnips, and winter squash, to name a few. Oats are extremely rich in soluble fiber; their bran makes a good addition to cereals and baked goods. Soluble fiber is also helpful in lowering elevated LDL cholesterol levels, a serious problem in many people with diabetes.

Fig

The leaves of the fig tree are a very useful blood-sugar-lowering treatment. Fig trees can be grown in warmer climates. Use caution if you are taking insulin or an oral hypoglycemic drug.

Flaxseed Oil

Supplements containing essential fatty acids, such as Flaxseed Oil, can help repair the cellular damage caused by a lifetime of high sugar consumption.

- Combine 4 oz. of cottage cheese with 1.5 oz. of flaxseed oil and 1 oz. of milk into a blender.

- Add honey or fresh fruits to add sweetness.

- Blend this mixture and drink daily each morning.

Garlic & Onions

Consume garlic and onions in large quantities. These flavorful foods help to lower 'bad' LDL cholesterol and raise 'good' HDL cholesterol and prevent heart disease. People with diabetes tend to have a greater risk of heart disease because the lack of insulin prompts fat to float throughout the bloodstream longer and in higher levels than normal. Eat a diet abundant in vegetables and moderate in sweet fruits to get a rich array of antioxidants such as vitamin C, the carotenes, and flavonoids. Antioxidants help prevent fats from oxidizing and causing damage to artery walls, which can lead to plaque build up and heart disease.

Green Tea

Green tea affects blood sugar by enhancing insulin in the body. Additionally, it inhibits the absorption of glucose in the intestines which prohibits peak levels of blood sugar.

Whole Foods

Whole foods such as fruits,vegetables, grains, beans, nuts, and seeds are rich in fiber and other nutritional factors that help stabilize blood sugar levels.

- Eat at least five fruits every day. Fruits like banana, blackberry, blueberries, cranberries, figs, grapefruit, pomegranate juice, granny smith apples, kiwi fruits, and citrus fruits are highly recommended.

Try to eat every color from whole foods each day to control high blood sugar levels. Excellent vegetables include artichoke, black beans, cabbage, carrots, cucumber, garlic, lettuce, onion, radish, string beans, tomatoes, spinach, squash, turnip, and brown rice.

Vitamin C

Studies have shown that certain anti-oxidants when taken with other supplements considered as natural cures for diabetes, has a good effect on diabetics by helping lower high sugar blood levels.

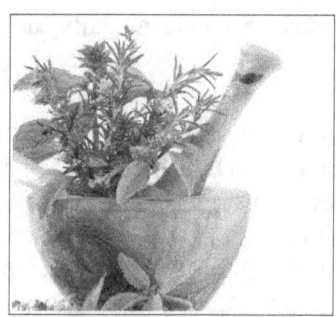

Foot Care

Diabetes mellitus (DM) represents several diseases in which high blood glucose levels over time can damage the nerves, kidneys, eyes, and blood vessels. Diabetes can also decrease the body's ability to fight infection. When diabetes is not well controlled, damage to the organs and impairment of the immune system is likely. Foot problems commonly develop in people with diabetes and can quickly become serious.

- With damage to the nervous system, a person with diabetes may not be able to feel his or her feet properly. Normal sweat secretion and oil production that lubricates the skin of the foot is impaired. These factors together can lead to abnormal pressure on the skin, bones, and joints of the foot during walking and can lead to breakdown of the skin of the foot. Sores may develop.

- Damage to blood vessels and impairment of the immune system from diabetes make it difficult to heal these wounds. Bacterial infection of the skin, connective tissues, muscles, and bones can then occur. These infections can develop into gangrene. Because of the poor blood flow, antibiotics cannot get to the site of the infection easily. Often, the only treatment for this is amputation of the foot or leg. If the infection spreads to the bloodstream, this process can be life-threatening.

- People with diabetes must be fully aware of how to prevent foot problems before they occur, to recognize problems early, and to seek the right treatment when problems do occur. Although treatment for diabetic foot problems has improved, prevention - including good control of blood sugar level - remains the best way to prevent diabetic complications.

- People with diabetes should learn how to examine their own feet and how to recognize the early signs and symptoms of diabetic foot problems.

- They should also learn what is reasonable to manage routine at home foot care, how to recognize when to call the doctor, and how to recognize when a problem has become serious enough to seek emergency treatment.

Causes

Several risk factors increase a person with diabetes chances of developing foot problems and diabetic infections in the legs and feet.

- *Footwear*: Poorly fitting shoes are a common cause of diabetic foot problems.
  - If the patient has red spots, sore spots, blisters, corns, calluses, or consistent pain associated with wearing shoes, new properly fitting footwear must be obtained as soon as possible.
  - If the patient has common foot abnormalities such as flat feet, bunions, or hammertoes, prescription shoes or shoe inserts may be necessary.

- *Nerve damage*: People with long-standing or poorly controlled diabetes are at risk for having damage to the nerves in their feet. The medical term for this is *peripheral neuropathy*.

  - Because of the nerve damage, the patient may be unable to feel their feet normally. Also, they may be unable to sense the position of their feet and toes while walking and balancing. With normal nerves, a person can usually sense if their shoes are rubbing on the feet or if one part of the foot is becoming strained while walking.

○ A person with diabetes may not properly sense minor injuries (such as cuts, scrapes, blisters), signs of abnormal wear and tear (that turn into calluses and corns), and foot strain. Normally, people can feel if there is a stone in their shoe, then remove it immediately. A person who has diabetes may not be able to perceive a stone. Its constant rubbing can easily create a sore.

• *Poor circulation*: Especially when poorly controlled, diabetes can lead to accelerated hardening of the arteries or atherosclerosis. When blood flow to injured tissues is poor, healing does not occur properly.

• *Trauma to the foot*: Any trauma to the foot can increase the risk for a more serious problem to develop.

• *Infections:*

○ Athlete's foot, a fungal infection of the skin or toenails, can lead to more serious bacterial infections and should be treated promptly.

○ Ingrown toenails should be handled right away by a foot specialist. Toenail fungus should also be treated.

• *Smoking*: Smoking any form of tobacco causes damage to the small blood vessels in the feet and legs. This damage can disrupt the healing process and is a major risk factor for infections and amputations. The importance of smoking cessation cannot be overemphasized.

Diabetes foot ulcers are the leading cause of amputations.

Symptoms

- Persistent pain can be a symptom of sprain, strain, bruise, overuse, improperly fitting shoes, or underlying infection.

- Redness can be a sign of infection, especially when surrounding a wound, or of abnormal rubbing of shoes or socks.

- Swelling of the feet or legs can be a sign of underlying inflammation or infection, improperly fitting shoes, or poor venous circulation. Other signs of poor circulation include the following:

  ○ Pain in the legs or buttocks that increases with walking but improves with rest (claudication)

  ○ Hair no longer growing on the lower legs and feet

  ○ Hard shiny skin on the legs

  ○ Localized warmth can be a sign of infection or inflammation, perhaps from wounds that won't heal or that heal slowly.

- Any break in the skin is serious and can result from abnormal wear and tear, injury, or infection. Calluses and corns may be a sign of chronic trauma to the foot. Toenail fungus, athlete's foot, and ingrown toenails may lead to more serious bacterial infections.

- Drainage of pus from a wound is usually a sign of infection. Persistent bloody drainage is also a sign of a potentially serious foot problem.

- A limp or difficulty walking can be sign of joint problems, serious infection, or improperly fitting shoes.

- Fever or chills in association with a wound on the foot can be a sign of a limb-threatening or life-threatening infection.

- Red streaking away from a wound or redness spreading out from a wound is a sign of a progressively worsening infection.

- New or lasting numbness in the feet or legs can be a sign of nerve damage from diabetes, which increases a persons risk for leg and foot problems.

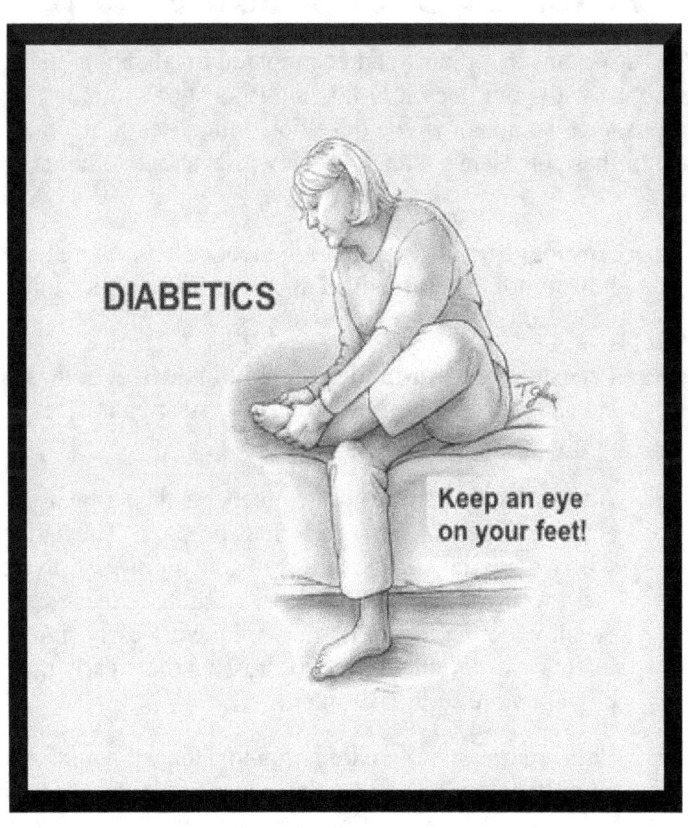

When to Seek Medical Care

Write down any symptoms and be prepared to talk about them on the phone with your doctor. Following is a list of common reasons to call a doctor if you develop a foot or leg problem. For most of these problems, a doctor visit within about 72 hours is best.

- Any **significant trauma** to the feet or legs, no matter how minor, needs medical attention. Even minor injuries can result in serious infections.

- Persistent **mild-to-moderate pain** in the feet or legs is a signal that something is wrong. Constant pain is never normal.

- Any new **blister, wound, or ulcer** less than 1 inch across can become a more serious problem. The patient will need to develop a plan with a doctor on how to treat these wounds. Any new areas of warmth, redness, or swelling on the feet or legs are frequently early signs of infection or inflammation. Addressing them early may prevent more serious problems.

- **Pain, redness, or swelling** around a toenail could mean an ingrown toenail - a leading cause of diabetic foot infections and amputations. Prompt and early treatment is essential.

- New or constant **numbness** in the feet or legs can be a sign of diabetic nerve damage (neuropathy) or of impaired circulation in the legs. Both conditions can put you at risk for serious problems such as infections and amputations.

- **Difficulty walking** can result from diabetic arthritis (Charcot's joints), often a sign of abnormal strain or pressure on the foot or of poorly fitting shoes. Early intervention is key to preventing more serious problems including falls as well as lower extremity skin breakdown and infections.

- Constant **itching** in the feet can be a sign of fungal infection or dry skin, both of which can lead to infection.

- **Calluses or corns** developing on the feet should be professionally removed. Home removal is not recommended.

- **Fever,** defined as a temperature over 98.6°F (37°C), in association with any other symptoms or even fever alone should prompt a call to a doctor's office. The degree of fever does not always correlate with the seriousness of infection. You could have no fever or a very low fever and still have a serious infection. Be especially cautious of fever.

Foot Care Treatment

Foot problems commonly develop in people with diabetes and can quickly become serious. When there is damage to the nervous system, a person with diabetes may not be able to feel his or her feet properly, even a stone in a shoe may not be detected which can result in an ulcer. Normal sweat secretion and oil production that lubricates the skin of the foot is impaired. These factors together can lead to abnormal pressure on the skin, bones, and joints of the foot during walking and can lead to breakdown of the skin of the foot.

It's important to learn how to avoid serious foot problems that can lead to a toe, foot, or leg amputation. There are a number of ways to prevent problems from developing with feet:

- check your feet every day. You may have serious foot problems, yet feel no pain. Check your feet for cuts, sores, red spots, swelling, and infected toenails. Make checking your feet part of your everyday routine. If you have trouble bending over to see your feet, use a mirror to help. You also can ask a family member or caregiver to help you. Make sure to call your doctor right away if a cut, sore, blister, or bruise on your foot does not begin to heal after one day

- wash your feet every day. Use warm, not hot, water with a mild soap. Before bathing or showering, test the water to make sure it is not too hot. You can use a thermometer (32°-35° C, 90° to 95° F is safe) or your elbow

- dry your feet well. Be sure to dry between your toes. Use talcum powder or cornstarch to keep the skin between your toes dry. Keep the skin soft and smooth by rubbing a thin coat of skin lotion, cream, or petroleum jelly on the tops and bottoms of your feet. Do not put lotion or cream between your toes as this might cause an infection

- smooth corns and calluses gently. Do not cut them. Don't use razor blades, corn plasters, or liquid corn and callus removers as they can damage your skin. If you have corns and calluses, check with your doctor or foot care specialist about the best way to care for them

- trim your toenails weekly or when needed. Trim toenails straight across and smooth them with an emery board or nail file. Don't cut into the corners of the toenail. If you can't see well, if your toenails are thick or yellowed, or if your nails curve and grow into the skin, have a foot care specialist trim them

- select the proper footwear. Wearing the right shoes is very important for preventing serious foot problems. Athletic or walking shoes are good for daily wear as they support your feet and allow them to breathe. Never wear vinyl or plastic shoes, because they don't stretch or breathe. When buying shoes make sure they are comfortable from the start and have enough room for your toes. Don't buy shoes with pointed toes or high heels as they put too much pressure on your toes

- do not walk bare foot - not even indoors as it is easy to step on something and hurt your feet

- along with shoes that fit well and protect your feet, always wear socks, stockings, or nylons with your shoes to help avoid blisters and sores. Choose clean, lightly padded socks that fit well. Socks that have no seams are best

- check the insides of your shoes before you put them on to be sure the lining is smooth and that there are no objects in them. You may need special shoes or shoe inserts to prevent serious foot problems

- protect your feet from hot and cold. Wear shoes at the beach or on hot pavement. Put sunscreen on the top of your feet to prevent sunburn. Keep your feet away from radiators and open fires

- do not put hot water bottles or heating pads on your feet. Wear socks at night if your feet get cold

- lined boots are good in winter to keep your feet warm. Check your feet often in cold weather to avoid frostbite

- wiggle your toes for five minutes, two or three times a day. Move your ankles up and down and in and out to improve blood flow in your feet and legs. Don't cross your legs for long periods of time

- don't wear tight socks, elastic or rubber bands, or garters around your legs

- be more active. Ask your health care provider to help plan a daily activity program that is right for you. Walking, dancing, swimming, and bicycling are good forms of exercise that are easy on the feet. Wear athletic shoes that fit well and that provide good support. Avoid activities that are hard on the feet, such as running and jumping

Antibiotics: If the doctor determines that a wound or ulcer on the patient's feet or legs is infected, or if the wound has high a risk of becoming infected, such as a cat bite, antibiotics will be prescribed to treat the infection or the potential infection. It is very important that the patient take the entire course of antibiotics as prescribed. Generally, the patient should see some improvement in the wound in two to three days and may see improvement the first day. For limb-threatening or life-threatening infections, the patient will be admitted to the hospital and given IV antibiotics. Less serious infections may be treated with pills as an outpatient. The doctor may give a single dose of antibiotics as a shot or IV dose prior to starting pills in the clinic or emergency department.

Referral to wound care center: Many of the larger community hospitals now have wound care centers specializing in the treatment of diabetic lower extremity wounds and ulcers along with other difficult-to-treat wounds. In these multi-disciplinary centers, professionals of many specialties including doctors, nurses, and therapists work with the patient and their doctor in developing a treatment plan for the wound or leg ulcer. Treatment plans may include surgical debridement of the wound, improvement of circulation through surgery or therapy, special dressings, and antibiotics. The plan may include a combination of treatments.

Referral to podiatrist or orthopedic surgeon: If the patient has bone-related problems, toenail problems, corns and calluses, hammertoes, bunions, flat feet, heel spurs, arthritis, or have difficulty with finding shoes that fit, a physician may refer you to one of these specialists. They create shoe inserts, prescribe shoes, remove calluses and have expertise in surgical solutions for bone problems. They can also be an excellent resource for how to care for the patient's feet routinely.

Home health care: The patient's doctor may prescribe a home health nurse or aide to help with wound care and dressings, monitor blood sugar, and help the patient take antibiotics and other medications properly during the healing period.

Where to Get More Help with Your Diabetes

People Who Can Help You

Your doctor.

You may see your regular doctor for diabetes care or someone who has special training in caring for people with diabetes. A doctor with special training in diabetes is called an endocrinologist or diabetologist.

You'll talk with your doctor about what kind of medicines you need and how much you should take. You'll also agree on a target blood glucose range and blood pressure and cholesterol targets. Your doctor will do tests to be sure your blood glucose, blood pressure, and cholesterol are staying on track and you're staying healthy. Ask your doctor if you should take aspirin every day to help prevent heart disease.

Your diabetes educator.

A diabetes educator may be a nurse, a dietitian, or another kind of health care worker. Diabetes educators teach you about meal planning, diabetes medicines, physical activity, how to check your blood glucose, and how to fit diabetes care into your everyday life. Be sure to ask questions if you don't understand something.

Your family and friends.

Taking care of your diabetes is a daily job. You may need help or support from your family or friends. You may want to bring a family member or close friend with you when you visit your doctor or diabetes educator. Taking good care of your diabetes can be a family affair!

A counsellor or mental health worker.

You might feel sad about having diabetes or get tired of taking care of yourself. Or you might be having problems because of work, school, or family. If diabetes makes you feel sad or angry, or if you have other problems that worry you, you can talk with a counsellor or mental health worker. Your doctor or diabetes educator can help you find a counsellor.

Canadian Diabetes Association
1400-522 University Ave
Toronto ON M5G 2R5
General Inquiries 416-363-3373.
Phone: 1-800 BANTING (226-8464)
Email: info@diabetes.ca

American Diabetes Association
1701 North Beauregard Street
Alexandria, VA 22311
Phone: 1-800-DIABETES (800-342-2383)

Diabetes UK Central Office
Macleod House,
10 Parkway,
London NW1 7AA
Phone: 0345 123 2399
Fax: 020 7424 1001
Email: info@diabetes.org.uk

FOOD SUBSTITUTE LIST

FOOD	SUBSTITUTE
Bacon	Back bacon (Canadian bacon), turkey bacon, smoked turkey or lean prosciutto (Italian ham)
Beef, pork, veal, lamb	Lean cuts trimmed of all visible fat, or substitute with chicken or turkey without the skin
Bologna, salami, or corned beef	Lean ham, low-fat cold cuts, or sliced turkey breast
Bread crumbs, dry	Rolled oats or crushed bran cereal
Bread, white	Whole-grain bread
Butter	Lower calorie, soft margarine, vegetable cooking sprays, or non-stick cookware 1 tablespoon butter = 1 tablespoon soft margarine (low in saturated fat and 0 grams trans fat) or 3/4 tablespoon vegetable oil
Butter, margarine, shortening, or oil in baked goods	Applesauce or prune puree for half of the called-for butter, shortening or oil; butter spreads or shortenings specially formulated for baking without trans fats *Note: To avoid dense, soggy or flat baked goods, don't substitute oil for butter or shortening. Also don't substitute diet, whipped or tub-style margarine for regular margarine.*
Butter, margarine, shortening or oil to prevent sticking	Cooking spray or non-stick pans
Cheese, (American, Cheddar, Swiss)	Cheeses with 5 or less grams of fat per ounce (e.g. reduced-fat, low-fat or fat-free). Reduced-fat is easier to substitute when cooking
Chocolate chips or nuts	Raisins or dried fruit

FOOD	SUBSTITUTE
Condensed cream soup	99% fat-free condensed cream soup
Cream	Fat-free half-and-half, evaporated skim milk; 1 cup heavy cream = 1 cup evaporated skim milk, or 1/2 cup low-fat yogurt and 1/2 cup plain low-fat unsalted cottage cheese
Cream cheese	Light, fat-free products, or Neufchatel cheese; 4 tablespoons soft margarine (low in saturated fat and 0 grams *trans* fat) blended with 1 cup dry, unsalted low-fat cottage cheese; add a small amount of fat-free milk if needed
Creamed Cottage cheese	Non-fat or 1% fat cottage cheese, or farmer's cheese
Creamed soup	Fat-free milk-based soups, mashed potato flakes, or pureed carrots, potatoes or tofu for thickening agents
Desserts: cakes or pastries	Angel food cake, fruit, gelatin
Egg noodles	Noodles made without egg yolk
Eggs	Two egg whites or 1/4 cup egg substitute for each whole egg
Flour, all-purpose	Whole-wheat flour for half of the all-purpose flour needed in baked goods *Note: Whole-wheat pastry flour is less dense and works well in softer products like cakes and muffins.* *TIP: Use a can of Black Beans, drained and rinsed, when making brownies. This cuts the gluten and gives an extra bit of protein.* *1 cup flour = 1 cup black bean puree (15 oz. Can)*

FOOD	SUBSTITUTE
Fried chicken	Oven baked or grilled chicken
Fruit canned in heavy syrup	Fruit canned in its own juices or in water, or fresh fruit
Frying	Broil, bake, microwave, poach, steam, grill, stir fry
Gravy	Gravies made with broth and thickened with flour or cornstarch
Ground beef	Extra-lean or lean ground beef, ground chicken breast or turkey breast (make sure no poultry skin has been added to the product)
Ice cream	Ices, sorbet, low-fat or reduced-fat ice cream, frozen yogurt
Lettuce, iceberg	Arugula, chicory, collard greens, dandelion greens, kale, mustard greens, spinach or watercress
Margarine, regular	Lower calorie margarine in tubs, vegetable cooking sprays, or non-stick cookware.
Mayonnaise	Reduced-fat, cholesterol free, low-fat, or fat-free *Note: If making a dip, substitute plain nonfat or low fat yogurt. Reduce the amount required in the recipe.*
Meat as the main ingredient	Use three times as many vegetables as the meat on pizzas or in casseroles, soups and stews
Milk, evaporated	Evaporated skim milk
Milk, whole	Reduced-fat or fat-free milk
Mozzarella cheese	Part-skim mozzarella cheese

FOOD	SUBSTITUTE
Oil for sautéing	Water, broth, tomato juice
Oil-based marinades	Wine, balsamic vinegar, fruit juice or fat-free broth
Pasta, enriched (white)	Whole-wheat pasta
Rice, white	Brown rice, wild rice, bulgur rice, or pearl barley
Ricotta cheese	Non-fat, lite, or part-skim
Salad dressing	Reduced-fat, cholesterol free, low-fat, or fat-free dressings; or lemon juice, vinegar, or mustard - reduce the amount required in the recipe
Salt	Herbs, spices, citrus juices (lemon, lime, orange), rice vinegar, salt-free seasoning mixes or herb blends; Reduce by 1/2 or eliminate
Seasoning salt, such as garlic salt, celery salt or onion salt	Herb-only seasonings, such as garlic powder, celery seed or onion flakes; or use finely chopped herbs or garlic, celery or onions
Short ribs	Grilled or baked salmon, grilled lean beef tenderloin
Soups, sauces, dressings, crackers, or canned meat, fish or vegetables	Low-sodium or reduced-sodium versions
Sour cream	Low-fat unsalted cottage cheese plus low-fat or fat-free yogurt; or just use fat-free sour cream
Soy sauce	Sweet-and-sour sauce, hot mustard sauce or low-sodium soy sauce
Sugar	In most baked goods you can reduce the amount of sugar by one-half; intensify sweetness by adding vanilla, nutmeg, cinnamon, stevia, honey, maple syrup, or beet sugar
Syrup	Pureed fruit, such as applesauce, or low-calorie, sugar-free syrup

FOOD	SUBSTITUTE
Tuna, packed in oil	Tuna, packed in water
Unsweetened baking chocolate (1 ounce)	3 tablespoons unsweetened cocoa powder or carob powder plus 1 tablespoon vegetable oil or soft margarine; since carob is sweeter than cocoa, reduce the sugar in the recipe by 25%
Whipped cream	Chilled evaporated skim milk, whipped
Whole milk or 2% milk	1% milk or skim milk
Yogurt, fruit-flavored	Plain low-fat yogurt with fresh fruit slices

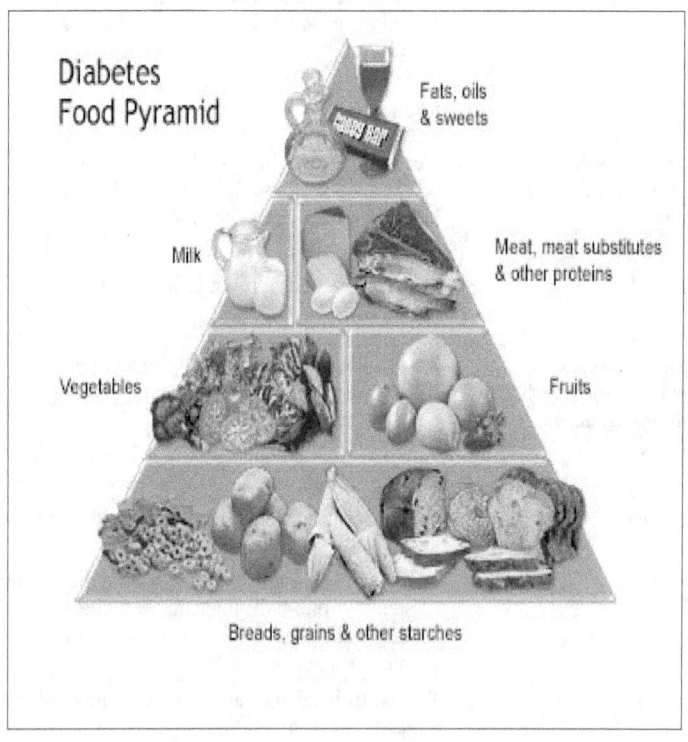

Diabetes Food Pyramid

Fats, oils & sweets

Milk

Meat, meat substitutes & other proteins

Vegetables

Fruits

Breads, grains & other starches

Diabetic Friendly Recipes

Quiche For Only You

Ingredients
> 1/3 cup chopped fresh mushrooms
> 1 teaspoon butter
> 1 egg
> 3 tablespoons 2% milk
> 1/8 teaspoon pepper
> Dash ground nutmeg
> 1/4 cup shredded Swiss cheese
> 1 teaspoon real bacon bits
> 1 teaspoon minced chives

Directions

1. In a small skillet, saute the mushrooms in butter until softened.

2. In a small bowl, beat egg, milk, pepper and nutmeg.

3. Stir in the mushrooms, cheese, bacon and chives.

4. Pour into a 5-in. pie plate coated with cooking spray.

5. Bake at 350° for 30 minutes or until set. Let stand for 5 minutes before serving.

Feta Frittata
Serves 2

Ingredients
> 1 green onion, thinly sliced
> 1 small garlic clove, minced
> 2 eggs
> 1/2 cup egg substitute

4 tablespoons crumbled feta cheese, divided
1/3 cup chopped plum tomato
4 thin slices peeled avocado
2 tablespoons reduced-fat sour cream

Directions

1. Heat a 6-in. nonstick skillet coated with cooking spray over medium heat.
2. Saute onion and garlic until tender. Whisk the eggs, egg substitute and 3 tablespoons feta cheese.
3. Add egg mixture to skillet (mixture should set immediately at edges). Cover and cook for 4-6 minutes or until nearly set.
4. Sprinkle with tomato and remaining feta cheese.
5. Cover and cook 2-3 minutes longer or until eggs are completely set.
6. Let stand for 5 minutes. Cut in half; serve with avocado and sour cream.

Fruity Granola
9 cups

Ingredients
> 5 cups old-fashioned oats
> 1 cup sliced almonds
> 1/2 cup sunflower kernels
> 1/2 cup ground flaxseed
> 1/2 cup packed brown sugar
> 1/4 cup maple syrup
> 1/4 cup honey
> 2 tablespoons canola oil
> 1/2 teaspoon salt
> 1/2 teaspoon ground cinnamon
> 1 teaspoon vanilla extract
> 1/2 cup dried cranberries
> 1/2 cup dried banana chips
> 1/2 cup dried apricots, halved

Directions

1. In a large bowl, combine the oats, almonds, sunflower kernels and flax.
2. In a small saucepan, combine the brown sugar, maple syrup, honey, oil, salt and cinnamon.
3. Cook and stir over medium heat for 2-3 minutes or until brown sugar is dissolved and mixture is heated through.
4. Remove from the heat; stir in vanilla.
5. Pour over oat mixture and toss to coat.
6. Transfer to a 15-in. x 10-in. x 1-in. baking pan coated with cooking spray.
7. Bake at 350° for 20-25 minutes or until golden brown, stirring every 8 minutes.
8. Cool completely on a wire rack.
9. Stir in dried fruits.
10. Store in an airtight container.

Fruit Salad with Vanilla
Serves 10

Ingredients
> 1 pound fresh strawberries, quartered
> 1-1/2 cups seedless red and/or green grapes, halved
> 2 medium bananas, sliced
> 2 kiwifruit, peeled, sliced and quartered
> 1 cup cubed fresh pineapple
> 1 can (21 ounces) peach pie filling
> 3 teaspoons vanilla extract

Directions
> In a large bowl, combine the strawberries, grapes, bananas, kiwi and pineapple. Fold in pie filling and vanilla. Chill until serving.

Honey Grapefruit and Bananas

Ingredients

1 (24-ounce) jar refrigerated red grapefruit sections
1 cup sliced banana
1 tablespoon fresh chopped mint
1 tablespoon honey

Directions

1. Drain grapefruit sections, reserving 1/4 cup juice.
2. Combine grapefruit sections, juice, and remaining ingredients in a medium bowl.
3. Toss gently to coat.
4. Serve immediately, or cover and chill.

Springtime Cereal
Serves 2

Ingredients

3/4 cup wheat and barley nugget cereal
1/4 cup 100% bran cereal
2 teaspoons toasted sunflower seeds
2 teaspoons toasted sliced almonds
1 tablespoon raisins
1/2 cup bananas, sliced
1 cup strawberries, sliced
1 cup low-fat raspberry or strawberry yogurt

Directions

1. Mix the wheat and barley nugget cereal, bran cereal, sunflower seeds, and almonds in a medium bowl.
2. Add the raisins, the bananas, and half of the strawberries.
3. Gently stir in the yogurt and divide between 2 bowls.
4. Scatter the remaining strawberries over the top.

Cinnamon French Toast
Serves 2

Ingredients
>4 slices cinnamon bread
>4 egg whites or equivalent egg substitute
>1 teaspoon vanilla extract
>1/8 teaspoon nutmeg cinnamon
>Powdered sugar
>Syrup

Directions
1. Spray pan with non-stick spray.
2. Crack egg whites into a bowl, discarding the yolks.
3. Add vanilla and nutmeg. Whip well.
4. Dip bread into egg mixture, coating both sides.
5. Over medium heat, toast bread.
6. Sprinkle cinnamon on each side of the bread. When done, sprinkle with powdered sugar and serve.
7. If desired, top with syrup.

Strawberry Yogurt Breakfast Split
Serves 1

Ingredients
>1 banana
>1 cup fresh strawberries
>1/2 cup vanilla yogurt
>1 tablespoon toasted almonds, chopped

Directions
1. Peel and split banana.
2. Place banana halves in serving bowl.
3. Top with strawberries, yogurt, and almonds.

Cantaloupe Delight
Serves 4

Ingredients
 1/2 cantaloupe
 1 cup fat free milk
 1-1/2 cups ice
 1 to 2 teaspoons sugar or sweetener

Directions
 1. Cut cantaloupe into small cubes.
 2. Blend all ingredients until smooth.
 3. Sweeten to taste.

Spanish Omelet
Serves 5

Ingredients
 5 small potatoes, peeled and sliced
 1 teaspoon olive oil or
 vegetable cooking spray
 1/2 medium onion, minced
 1 small zucchini, sliced
 1-1/2 cup green/red peppers, sliced thin
 5 medium mushrooms, sliced
 3 whole eggs, beaten
 5 egg whites, beaten
 3 ounces shredded part-skim mozzarella cheese
 1 tablespoon parmesan cheese
 Pepper, garlic salt, and herbs to taste

Directions
 1. Preheat the oven to 375° F.
 2. Cook potatoes in boiling water until tender.
 3. In a nonstick pan, add oil or vegetable spray and warm at medium heat.
 4. Add the onion and sauté until brown.
 5. Add vegetables and sauté until tender but not brown.

6. In a medium mixing bowl, slightly beat the eggs and egg whites, pepper, garlic salt, and mozzarella cheese.
7. Stir egg cheese mixture into the cooked vegetables.
8. Oil or spray a 10-inch pie pan or ovenproof skillet.
9. Transfer potatoes and eggs mixture to pan.
10. Spread with parmesan cheese and bake omelet until firm and brown on top, about 20 to 30 minutes.

Homestyle Biscuits
Serves 15

Ingredients
    2 cups flour
    2 teaspoons baking powder
    1/4 teaspoon baking soda
    1/4 teaspoon salt
    2 tablespoons sugar
    2/3 cup 1% buttermilk
    3 tablespoons + 1 teaspoon vegetable oil

Directions
1. Preheat the oven to 450° F.
2. In a medium bowl, combine flour, baking powder, baking soda, salt and sugar.
3. In a small bowl, stir together butter milk and oil. Pour over flour mixture; stir until well mixed.
4. On a lightly floured surface, knead dough gently for 10 to 20 strokes.
5. Roll or pat dough to 3/4 inch thickness.
6. Cut with a 2-inch biscuit or cookie cutter, dipping cutter in flour between cuts.
7. Transfer biscuits to an ungreased sheet.
8. Bake for 12 minutes or until golden brown. Serve warm

Apple Coffee Cake
Serves 20

Ingredients
>5 cups tart apples, cored, peeled chopped
>1 cup sugar
>1 cup dark raisins
>1/2 cup pecans, chopped
>1/4 cup vegetable oil
>2 teaspoons vanilla
>1 cup egg, beaten
>2-1/2 cups sifted all-purpose flour
>1-1/2 teaspoon baking soda
>2 teaspoons ground cinnamon

Directions
1. Preheat oven to 350° F.
2. Lightly oil a 13x9x2 inch pan.
3. In a large mixing bowl, combine apples with sugar, raisins, and pecans; mix well. Let stand 30 minutes.
4. Stir in oil, vanilla, and eggs.
5. Sift together flour, baking soda, and cinnamon; stir into apple mixture about 1/3 at a time just enough to moisten dry ingredients.
6. Turn batter into pan. Bake 35 to 40 minutes. Cool cake slightly before serving.

●●●

Broccoli Cheddar Bake
Serves 6

Ingredients
>   4 cups chopped fresh broccoli
>   1/2 cup finely chopped onion
>   2 tablespoons water
>   1 1/2 cups egg substitute
>   1 cup fat-free milk
>   1 cup shredded cheddar cheese
>   1/2 teaspoon ground black pepper

Directions
1. Preheat the oven to 350 F.
2. Lightly coat a baking dish with cooking spray.
3. In a nonstick skillet, combine the broccoli, onion and water.
4. Saute over medium-high heat until the vegetables are tender, about 5 to 8 minutes.
5. Keep adding water to prevent the vegetables from drying out, but use as little water as possible.
6. Drain and set aside when the broccoli is done.
7. In a bowl, combine the egg substitute, milk and 3/4 cup cheese.
8. Add in the broccoli mixture and pepper. Stir to mix well.
9. Transfer the mixture into the prepared baking dish.
10. Set the baking dish into a large pan filled with about 1 inch of water.
11. Bake uncovered until a knife inserted in the center comes out clean, about 45 minutes.
12. Remove from the oven and top with the remaining 1/4 cup shredded cheese.
13. Let stand about 10 minutes before serving.

Chicken with Asparagus and Penne
Serves 2

Ingredients
>1-1/2 cups uncooked whole-grain penne pasta
>1 cup asparagus, cut into 1-inch pieces
>6 ounces boneless, skinless chicken breasts, cut into 1-inch cubes
>2 cloves garlic, minced
>1 can (14.5 ounces) diced tomatoes, no salt added, including juice
>2 teaspoons dried basil or oregano
>1 ounce soft goat cheese, crumbled
>1 tablespoon Parmesan cheese

Directions
1. Fill a large pot 3/4 full with water and bring to a boil.
2. Add the pasta and cook until al dente (tender), 10 to 12 minutes, or according to the package directions.
3. Drain the pasta thoroughly. Set aside.
4. In a pot fitted with a steamer basket, bring 1 inch of water to a boil.
5. Add the asparagus. Cover and steam until tender-crisp, about 2 to 3 minutes.
6. Spray a large nonstick frying pan with cooking spray.
7. Add the chicken and garlic and saute over medium-high heat.
8. Cook until the chicken is golden brown, about 5 to 7 minutes.
9. Add the tomatoes, including their juice, basil or oregano and simmer 1 minute more.
10. In a large bowl, add the cooked pasta, steamed asparagus, chicken mixture and goat cheese.
11. Toss gently to mix evenly.
12. To serve, divide the pasta mixture between 2 plates.
13. Sprinkle each serving with 1/2 tablespoon Parmesan cheese.
14. Serve immediately.

Cod with Lemon and Capers
Serves 4

Ingredients
>   4 cod fillets, each 6 ounces
>   2 lemons
>   1 teaspoon low-sodium chicken-flavored bouillon
>   granules
>   1 cup hot tap water
>   1 tablespoon soft butter
>   1 tablespoon all-purpose (plain) flour
>   4 teaspoons capers, rinsed and drained

Directions
1. Preheat the oven to 350 F.
2. Spray 4 squares of foil with cooking spray.
3. Place 1 cod fillet on each of the foil squares.
4. Cut 1 lemon in half. Squeeze the juice from the lemon half over the fish.
5. Cut the other half of lemon into slices, place over the fish and seal the foil.
6. Place in the oven and bake until the fish is opaque throughout when tested with the tip of a knife, about 20 minutes.
7. While the fish is cooking, remove the peel from the second lemon. Take care to cut only the peel and not the pith. Slice the peel into 1/4-inch-wide strips. Set aside.
8. In a small bowl, add the chicken bouillon granules and the hot tap water. Stir until the granules dissolve. Set aside.
9. In another small bowl, mix the butter and flour together.
10. Transfer to a heavy saucepan. Stir over moderate heat until the butter-flour mixture melts.
11. Add the bouillon to the butter mixture and continue to stir until thickened.
12. Add the capers and remove from the heat.
13. Serve over the fish and garnish with the lemon peel.

Vegetable Quesadillas
Serves 4

Ingredients
>   1 large carrot, grated
>   1 zucchini, grated
>   8 flour tortillas
>   3/4 cup crumbled queso fresco or shredded Monterey
>   Jack cheese
>   Bottled hot sauce to taste

Directions
1. In a small bowl, mix carrot and zucchini.
2. Sprinkle 1/2 cup vegetable mixture over each of the four tortillas.
3. Top each tortilla with 3 tablespoons cheese.
4. Sprinkle with hot sauce, to taste.
5. Cover with a second tortilla.
6. Heat a nonstick pan over medium heat until hot.
7. Place each quesadilla in pan. Cook 1 minute. Turn over and cook 1 minute longer or until hot and cheese melts.
8. Cut each quesadilla into four quarters. Serve.

Chicken Vegetable Soup
Makes 6 servings

Ingredients
>   4 cups chicken broth
>   1/2 onion, chopped
>   1/2 teaspoon each basil, oregano, marjoram
>   1 clove garlic, minced
>   1/4 teaspoon pepper
>   2 cups assorted vegetables, chopped or 1x10-oz. bag
>   frozen vegetables
>   2 cups chicken, cooked & cubed
>   1-15 oz. can low sodium tomatoes

Directions
1. In a large saucepan, mix chicken broth, onions, herbs, garlic and pepper.
2. Stir in vegetables.
3. Bring to a boil.
4. Reduce heat, cover and simmer for 6-8 minutes or until vegetables are crisp-tender.
5. Stir in chicken and undrained tomatoes. Heat through.

Tortilla Roll-Ups
4 wraps

Ingredients
    4 whole wheat tortillas, 8-inch size
    1/4 cup low-fat cream cheese, softened
    12 slices (1 oz. each) lean turkey
    spinach leaves, washed and dried
    1 cup grated carrots

Directions
1. Spread about 1 tablespoon cream cheese on each tortilla, making sure to reach the edges.
2. Place 3 slices of meat on each tortilla.
3. Cover meat with spinach leaves and 1/4 cup grated carrots.
4. Roll tortilla tightly; secure with a toothpick if desired.

Spanish Omelet
Total Servings 5

Ingredients
    5 small potatoes, peeled and sliced
    Vegetable cooking spray
    1/2 medium onion, minced
    1 small zucchini, sliced
    1-1/2 cups green/red peppers, sliced thin
    5 medium mushrooms, sliced
    3 whole eggs, beaten
    5 egg whites, beaten

Pepper and garlic salt with herbs, to taste
3 ounces shredded part-skim mozzarella cheese
1 tablespoon low-fat parmesan cheese

Directions
1. Preheat oven to 375 °F.
2. Cook potatoes in boiling water until tender.
3. In a nonstick pan, add vegetable spray and warm at medium heat.
4. Add onion and sauté until brown.
5. Add vegetables and sauté until tender but not brown.
6. In a medium mixing bowl, slightly beat eggs and egg whites, pepper, garlic salt, and low-fat mozzarella cheese.
7. Stir egg-cheese mixture into the cooked vegetables.
8. In a 10-inch pie pan or ovenproof skillet, add vegetable spray and transfer potatoes and egg mixture to pan.
9. Sprinkle with low-fat parmesan cheese and bake until firm and brown on top, about 20–30 minutes.
10. Remove omelet from oven, cool for 10 minutes, and cut into five pieces.

Caribbean Red Snapper
Serves 4

Ingredients
2 tablespoons olive oil
1 medium onion, chopped
1/2 cup red pepper, chopped
1/2cup carrots, cut into strips
1 clove garlic, minced
1/2 cup dry white wine
3/4 pound red snapper fillet
1 large tomato, chopped
2 tablespoons pitted ripe olives, chopped
2 tablespoons crumbled low-fat feta or low-fat ricotta cheese

Directions
1. In a large skillet, heat olive oil over medium heat.
2. Add onion, red pepper, carrots, and garlic.
3. Sauté mixture for 10 minutes.
4. Add wine and bring to boil.
5. Push vegetables to one side of the pan.
6. Arrange fillets in a single layer in center of skillet.
7. Cover and cook for 5 minutes.
8. Add tomato and olives. Top with cheese.
9. Cover and cook for 3 minutes or until fish is firm but moist.
10. Transfer fish to serving platter.
11. Garnish with vegetables and pan juices.

Two Chesse Pizza
8 slices

Ingredients
- 2 tablespoons whole wheat flour
- 1 can (10 ounces) refrigerated pizza crust
- Vegetable cooking spray
- 2 tablespoons olive oil
- 1/2 cup low-fat ricotta cheese
- 1/2 teaspoon dried basil
- 1 small onion, minced
- 2 cloves garlic, minced
- 1/4 teaspoon salt (optional)
- 4 ounces shredded part-skim mozzarella cheese
- 2 cups mushrooms, chopped
- 1 large red pepper, cut into strips

Directions
1. Preheat oven to 425 °F.
2. Spread whole wheat flour over working surface.
3. Roll out dough with rolling pin to desired crust thickness.
4. Coat cookie sheet with vegetable cooking spray.
5. Transfer pizza crust to cookie sheet.
6. Brush olive oil over crust.

7. Mix low-fat ricotta cheese with dried basil, onion, garlic, and salt.
8. Spread this mixture over crust.
9. Sprinkle crust with part-skim mozzarella cheese.
10. Top cheese with mushrooms and red pepper.
11. Bake at 425 °F for 13-15 minutes or until cheese melts and crust is deep golden brown.
12. Cut into 8 slices.

Rice with Chicken, Spanish Style

Serves 8

Ingredients
>   2 tablespoons olive oil
>   2 medium onions, chopped
>   6 cloves garlic, minced
>   2 stalks celery, diced
>   2 medium red/green peppers, cut into strips
>   1 cup mushrooms, chopped
>   2 cups uncooked whole grain rice
>   3 pounds boneless chicken breast, cut into bite-sized pieces, skin removed
>   1-1/2 teaspoon salt (optional)
>   2-1/2 low-fat chicken broth
>   3 medium tomatoes, chopped
>   1 cup frozen peas
>   1 cup frozen corn
>   1 cup frozen green beans
>   Olives or capers for garnish (optional)

Directions
1. Heat olive oil over medium heat in a non-stick pot.
2. Add onion, garlic, celery, red/green pepper, and mushrooms.
3. Cook over medium heat, stirring often, for 3 minutes or until tender.
4. Add whole grain rice and sauté for 2–3 minutes, stirring constantly to mix all ingredients.
5. Add chicken, salt, chicken broth, water, and tomatoes.

6. Bring water to a boil.
7. Reduce heat to medium-low, cover, and let the casserole simmer until water is absorbed and rice is tender, about 20 minutes.
8. Stir in peas, corn, and beans and cook for 8–10 minutes.
9. When everything is hot, the casserole is ready to serve.
10. Garnish with olives or capers, if desired.

Pozole
8 servings

Ingredients
> 2 pounds lean beef, cubed (or, skinless, boneless chicken breasts)
> 1 tablespoon olive oil
> 1 large onion, chopped
> 1 clove garlic, finely chopped
> 1/4 teaspoon salt teaspoon pepper
> 1/4 cup fresh cilantro, chopped
> 1 can (15 ounces) stewed tomatoes
> 2 ounces tomato paste
> 1 can hominy

Directions
1. In a large pot, heat olive oil.
2. Add beef and sauté.
3. Add onion, garlic, salt, pepper, cilantro, and enough water to cover meat. Stir to mix ingredients evenly.
4. Cover pot and cook over low heat until meat is tender.
5. Add tomatoes and tomato paste.
6. Continue cooking for about 20 minutes.
7. Add hominy and continue cooking another 15 minutes, stirring occasionally. If too thick, add water for desired consistency.

Avocado Tacos

Ingredients

    1 medium onion, cut into thin strips
    2 large green peppers, cut into thin strips
    2 large red peppers, cut into thin strips
    1 cup fresh cilantro, finely chopped
    1 ripe avocado, peeled and seeded, cut into 12 slices
    1-1/2 cups fresh tomato salsa (see ingredients below)
    12 flour tortillas
    Vegetable cooking spray

Fresh Tomato Salsa Ingredients

    1 cup tomatoes, diced cup onions, diced
    1/2 clove garlic, minced
    2 teaspoon cilantro teaspoon jalapeño peppers, chopped
    1/2 teaspoon lime juice
    Pinch of cumin

Directions
1. Mix together all salsa ingredients and refrigerate in advance.
2. Coat skillet with vegetable spray.
3. Lightly sauté onion and green and red peppers.
4. Warm tortillas in oven and fill with peppers, onions, avocado, and salsa.
5. Fold tortillas and serve.
6. Top with cilantro.

Stir-Fried Beef and Chinese Vegetables
Serves 6

Ingredients

    2 tablespoons dry red wine
    1 tablespoons soy sauce
    1/2 teaspoon sugar
    1-1/2 teaspoon gingerroot, peeled, grated
    1lb boneless round steak, fat trimmed, cut across grain into 1-1/2 inch strips

2 tablespoons vegetable oil
2 medium onions, each cut into 8 wedges
1/2 lb fresh mushrooms, rinsed, trimmed, sliced
2 stalks (1/2 cup) celery, cut into 1/4 inch slices
2 small green peppers, cut into thin lengthwise strips
1 cup water chestnuts, drained, sliced
2 tablespoons cornstarch
1/4 cup water

Directions
1. Prepare marinade by mixing together wine, soy sauce, sugar, and ginger.
2. Marinate meat in mixture while preparing vegetables.
3. Heat 1 tablespoon oil in large skillet or wok.
4. Stir-fry onions and mushrooms for 3 minutes over medium-high heat.
5. Add celery and cook for 1 minute.
6. Add remaining vegetables and cook for 2 minutes or until green pepper is tender, but crisp.
7. Transfer vegetables to warm bowl.
8. Add remaining 1 tablespoon oil to skillet.
9. Stir-fry meat in oil for about 2 minutes, or until meat loses its pink color.
10. Blend cornstarch and water.
11. Stir into meat.
12. Cook and stir until thickened.
13. Return vegetables to skillet.
14. Stir gently and serve.

Scrumptious Meat Loaf
Serves 6

Inredients
1 lb ground beef, extra lean
1/2 cup (4oz) tomato paste
1/4 cup onion, chopped
1/4 cup green peppers
1/4 cup red peppers
1 cup tomatoes, fresh, blanched, chopped

1/2 teaspoon mustard, low sodium
1/4 teaspoon ground black pepper
1/2 teaspoon hot pepper, chopped
2 cloves garlic, chopped
2 stalks scallion, chopped
1/2 teaspoon ground ginger
1/8 teaspoon ground nutmeg
1 teaspoon orange rind, grated
1/2 teaspoon thyme, crushed
1/4 cup bread crumbs, finely grated

Directions
1. Mix all ingredients together
2. Place in 1-lb loaf pan (preferably with drip rack) and bake covered at 350° F for 50 minutes.
3. Uncover pan and continue baking for 12 minutes.

Barbecued Chicken
Serves 8

Ingredients
3 lb chicken parts (breast, drumstick, and thigh), skin and fat removed
1 large onion, thinly sliced
3 tablespoons vinegar
3 tablespoons Worcestershire sauce
Black pepper to taste
1 tablespoon hot pepper flakes
1 tablespoon chili powder
1 cup chicken stock or broth, fat skimmed from top

Directions
1. Place chicken in 13-by 9-by 2-inch pan.
2. Arrange onions over top.
3. Mix together vinegar, Worcestershire sauce, brown sugar, pepper, hot pepper flakes, chili powder, and stock.
4. Pour mixture over chicken and bake at 350° F for 1 hour or until done.
5. Baste occasionally.

20-Minute Chicken Creole
Serves 6

Ingredients
>4 medium chicken breast halves, skinless, boned, and cut
>into 1-inch strips
>1 cup (14 oz) tomatoes, cut up
>1 cup low-sodium chili sauce
>1 large green pepper, chopped
>1-1/2 cup celery, chopped
>1/4 cup onion, chopped
>2 cloves garlic, minced
>1 tablespoon fresh basil (or 1 teaspoon dried)
>1 tablespoon fresh parsley (1 teaspoon dried)
>1/4 teaspoon red pepper, crushed
>1/4 teaspoon salt
>Non-stick cooking spray

Directions
1. Spray deep skillet with nonstick cooking spray. Preheat pan over high heat.
2. Cook chicken in hot skillet, stirring, for 3-5 minutes or until no longer pink. Reduce heat.
3. Add tomatoes with juice, low sodium chili sauce, green pepper, celery, onion, garlic, basil, parsley, crushed red pepper, and salt.
4. Bring to boil and reduce heat. Simmer covered for 10 minutes.
5. Serve over hot cooked rice or whole wheat pasta

Salmon Dijon
Serves 6

Ingredients
>1 cup fat-free sour cream
>2 teaspoon dried dill
>3 tablespoons scallions, finely chopped
>2 tablespoons Dijon mustard

2 tablespoons lemon juice
10-1/2 lb salmon fillet with skin, cut in center
1/2 teaspoon garlic powder
1/2 teaspoon black pepper
As needed fat-free cooking spray

Directions
1. Whisk sour cream, dill, onion, mustard, and lemon juice in small bowl to blend.
2. Preheat oven to 400° F. Lightly oil baking sheet with cooking spray.
3. Place salmon, skin side down, on prepared sheet. Sprinkle with garlic powder and pepper, then spread with the sauce.
4. Bake salmon until just opaque in center, about 20 minutes.

Black Beans With Rice
Serves 6

Ingredients
1 lb black beans, dry
7 cup water
1 medium green pepper, coarsely chopped
1-1 cup onion, chopped
1-1/2 tablespoons vegetable oil
2 bay leaves
1 clove garlic, minced
1/2 teaspoon salt
1 tablespoons vinegar (or lemon juice)
6 cup rice, cooked in unsalted water
1 jar (4 oz) sliced pimento, drained
1 lemon, cut into wedges

Directions
1. Pick through beans to remove bad ones. Soak beans overnight in cold water. Drain and rinse.

2. In large soup pot or Dutch oven, stir together beans, water, green pepper, onion, oil, bay leaves, garlic, and salt. Cover and boil for 1 hour
3. Reduce heat and simmer, covered, for 3-4 hours or until beans are very tender. Stir occasionally, and add water if needed.
4. Remove and mash about a third of beans. Return to pot. Stir and heat through.
5. When ready to serve, remove bay leaves and stir in vinegar or lemon juice.
6. Serve over rice. Garnish with sliced pimento and lemon wedges.

Zucchini Lasagna
Serves 6

Ingredients
> 1/2 lb lasagna noodles, cooked in unsalted water
> 3/4 cup part-skim mozzarella cheese, grated
> 1-1/2 cup fat-free cottage cheese
> 1/4 cup Parmesan cheese, grated
> 1-1/2 cup raw zucchini, sliced
> 2-1/2 cup no salt added tomato sauce
> 2 teaspoon basil, dried
> 2 teaspoon oregano, dried
> 1/4 cup onion, chopped
> 1 clove garlic
> 1/8 teaspoon black pepper

Directions
1. Preheat oven to 350° F. Lightly spray 9-by 13 inch baking dish with vegetable oil spray.
2. In small bowl, combine 1/8 cup mozzarella and 1 tablespoons parmesan cheese. Set aside.
3. In medium bowl, combine remaining mozzarella and Parmesan cheese with all of the cottage cheese. Mix well and set aside.
4. Combine tomato sauce with remaining ingredients.

5. Spread thin layer of tomato sauce in bottom of baking dish.
6. Add 1/3 of noodles in single layer.
7. Spread 1/2 of cottage cheese mixture on top.
8. Add layer of zucchini.
9. Repeat layering.
10. Add thin coating of sauce.
11. Top with noodles, sauce, and reserved cheese mixture.
12. Cover with aluminum foil.
13. Bake for 30-40 minutes.
14. Cool for 10-15 minutes.
15. Cut into 6 portions.

Sweet and Sour Seashells
Serves 18

Ingredients
> 1 lb uncooked small seashell pasta (9 cups cooked)
> 2 tablespoons vegetable oil
> 3/4 cup sugar
> 1/2 cup cider vinegar
> 1/2 cup wine vinegar
> 1/2 cup water
> 3 tablespoons prepared mustard
> To taste black pepper
> 1 jar (2 oz) sliced pimentos
> 2 small cucumbers
> 2 small onions, thinly sliced
> 18 leaves lettuce

Directions
1. Cook pasta in unsalted water, drain, rinse with cold water, and drain again. Stir in oil.
2. Transfer to 4-quart bowl.
3. In blender, place sugar, vinegars, water, prepared mustard, salt, pepper, and pimento. Process at low speed for 15-20 seconds, or just enough so flecks of pimento can be seen.
4. Pour over pasta.

5. Score cucumber peel with fork tines. Cut cucumber in ½ lengthwise, then slice thinly. Add to pasta with onion slices. Toss well.
6. Marinate, covered, in refrigerator for 24 hours. Stir occasionally.
7. Drain, and serve on lettuce.

Fresh Cabbage and Tomato Salad
Serves 8

Ingredients
 1 head small cabbage, sliced thinly
 2 medium tomatoes, cut in cubes
 1 cup radishes, sliced
 1/4 teaspoon salt
 2 teaspoon olive oil
 2 tablespoons rice vinegar (or lemon juice)
 1/2 teaspoon black pepper
 1/2 teaspoon red pepper
 2 tablespoons fresh cilantro, chopped

Directions
 1. In large bowl, mix together cabbage, tomatoes, and radishes.
 2. In another bowl, mix together the rest of the ingredients and pour over vegetables.

Green Beans Sauté

Ingredients
 1 lb fresh or frozen green beans, cut in 1-inch pieces
 1 tablespoon vegetable oil
 1 large yellow onion, halved lengthwise, thinly sliced
 1/2 teaspoon salt
 1/8 teaspoon black pepper
 1 tablespoons fresh parsley, minced

Directions
1. If using fresh green beans, cook in boiling water for 10-12 minutes or steam for 2- 3 minutes until barely fork tender. Drain well. If using frozen green beans, thaw first.
2. Heat oil in large skillet. Sauté onion until golden.
3. Stir in green beans, salt, and pepper. Heat through.
4. Before serving, toss with parsley.

Italian Vegetable Bake

Ingredients
1 can (28 oz) tomatoes, whole
1 medium onion, sliced
1/2 lb fresh green beans, sliced
1/2 lb fresh okra, cut into
1/2-inch pieces (or 1/2 of 10-oz package frozen, cut)
3/4 cup green pepper, finely chopped
2 tablespoons lemon juice
1 tablespoon fresh basil, chopped, or 1 teaspoon dried basil, crushed
1-1/2 teaspoon fresh oregano leaves, chopped (or 1/2 teaspoon dried oregano, crushed)
3 medium (7-inch long) zucchini, cut into 1-inch cubes
1 medium eggplant, pared, cut into 1-inch cubes
2 tablespoons Parmesan cheese, grated

Directions
1. Drain and coarsely chop tomatoes. Save liquid.
2. Mix together tomatoes, reserved liquid, onion, green beans, okra, green pepper, lemon juice, and herbs.
3. Cover and bake at 325° F for 15 minutes.
4. Mix in zucchini and eggplant. t
5. Continue baking, covered, 60-70 minutes more or until vegetables are tender.
6. Sir occasionally.
7. Just before serving, sprinkle top with parmesan cheese.

Vegetable Stew

Ingredients
    3 cups water
    1 cube vegetable bouillon, low sodium
    2 cups white potatoes, cut in 2-inch strips
    2 cups carrots, sliced
    4 cups summer squash, cut in 1-inch squares
    1 cup summer squash, cut in 4 chunks
    1 can (15 oz) sweet corn, rinsed, drained (or 2 ears fresh corn, 1-1/2 cup)
    1 teaspoon thyme
    2 cloves garlic, minced
    1 stalk scallion, chopped
    1/2 small hot pepper, chopped
    1 cup onion, coarsely chopped
    1 cup tomatoes diced (add other favorite vegetables, such as broccoli and cauliflower)

Directions
1. Put water and bouillon in large pot and bring to a boil.
2. Add potatoes and carrots, and simmer for 5 minutes.
3. Add remaining ingredients, except for tomatoes, and continue cooking for 15 minutes over medium heat.
4. Remove four chunks of squash and puree in blender.
5. Return pureed mixture to pot and let cook for 10 minutes more.
6. Add tomatoes and cook for another 5 minutes.
7. Remove from flame and let sit for 10 minutes to allow stew to thicken.

Candied Yams

Ingredients
    3 medium yams
    1/4 cup brown sugar, packed
    1 teaspoon flour, sifted
    1/4 teaspoon salt
    1/4 teaspoon ground cinnamon

1/4 teaspoon ground nutmeg
1/4 teaspoon orange peel
1 teaspoon soft tub margarine
1/2 cup orange juice

Directions
1. Cut yams in half and boil until tender but firm (about 20 minutes). When cool enough to handle, peel and slice into 1/4-inch thickness.
2. Combine sugar, flour, salt, cinnamon, nutmeg, and grated orange peel.
3. Place 1/2 of sliced yams in medium-size casserole dish. Sprinkle with spiced sugar mixture.
4. Dot with 1/2 the amount of margarine.
5. Add second layer of yams, using the rest of the ingredients in the same order as above.
6. Add orange juice.
7. Bake uncovered for 20 minutes in oven that was preheated to 350° F.
8. Remove from flame and let sit for 10 minutes to allow stew to thicken.

Garlic Mashed Potatoes
Serves 6

Ingredients
2 large potatoes, peeled, quartered
2 cups skim milk
2 cloves garlic, large, chopped
1/2 teaspoon white pepper

Directions

To use sauce pan:

1. Cook potatoes, covered, in small amount of boiling water for 20-25 minutes or until tender.
2. Remove from heat. Drain and recover.

3. Meanwhile, in small saucepan over low heat, cook garlic in milk until soft (about 30 minutes).
4. Add milk-garlic mixture and white pepper to potatoes.
5. Beat with electric mixture on low speed, or mash, until smooth.

To use microwave:

1. Scrub potatoes, pat dry, and prick with fork.
2. On plate, cook potatoes uncovered on 100 percent (high) power until tender (about 12 minutes), turning over once. Let stand 5 minutes, then peel and quarter.
3. Meanwhile, in 4-cup measuring glass, combine milk and garlic.
4. Cook, uncovered, on 50 percent (medium) power until garlic is soft (about 45 minutes).
5. Continue as directed above.

Classic Macaroni and Cheese

Ingredients
    2 cups macaroni
    1/2 cup onions, chopped
    1/2 cup evaporated skim milk
    1 medium egg, beaten
    1/4 teaspoon black pepper
    1-1/4 cups (4 oz) low-fat sharp cheddar cheese finely shredded
    Non-stick cooking spray

Directions
1. Cook macaroni according to directions, but do not add salt to the cooking water. Drain and set aside. Spray casserole dish with nonstick cooking spray. Preheat oven to 350° F.
2. Lightly spray saucepan with nonstick cooking spray. Add onions and sauté for about 3 minutes.
3. In another bowl, combine macaroni, onions, and rest of ingredients and mix.
4. Transfer mixture into casserole dish.

5. Bake for 25 minutes, or until bubbly.
6. Let stand for 10 minutes before serving.

•••

Mango Shake
Serves 4

Ingredients
> 2 cups 1% milk
> 4 tablespoons frozen mango juice (or 1 fresh pitted mango)
> 1 small banana
> 2 ice cubes

Directions
> Put all ingredients into a blender. Blend until foamy. Serve immediately. Variations: Instead of mango, try orange juice, papaya, or strawberries.

Summer Breezes Smoothie
Serves 3

Ingredients
> 1 cup plain nonfat yogurt
> 6 medium strawberries
> 1 cup pineapple, crushed, canned in juice
> 1 medium banana
> 1 teaspoon vanilla extract
> 4 ice cubes

Directions
> Place all ingredients in a blender and purée until smooth.

1-2-3 Peach Cobbler
Serves 8

Ingredients
>1/2 teaspoon ground cinnamon
>1 tablespoon vanilla extract
>2 tablespoons cornstarch
>1 cup peach nectar
>1/4 cup pineapple juice or peach juice
>2 16-oz cans of peaches, sliced, packed in juice, drained
>(or 1 3/4 pounds fresh peaches)
>Nonstick cooking oil spray (to grease baking dish)
>1 tablespoon soft margarine
>1 cup dry pancake mix
>2/3 cup all-purpose flour
>1/2 cup sugar
>2/3 cup evaporated skim milk
>topping: 1/2 teaspoon nutmeg; 1 tablespoon brown sugar

Directions
1. Preheat oven to 400° F.
2. Combine cinnamon, vanilla, cornstarch, peach nectar, and pineapple or peach juice in a saucepan over medium heat. Stir constantly until mixture thickens and bubbles.
3. Add sliced peaches to mixture.
4. Reduce heat and simmer for 5 to 10 minutes.
5. In another saucepan, melt margarine and set aside.
6. Lightly spray an 8-inch square glass dish with cooking oil spray. Pour hot peach mixture into the dish.
7. In another bowl, combine pancake mix, flour, sugar, and melted margarine. Stir in milk.
8. Quickly spoon mixture over peach mixture.
9. Combine nutmeg and brown sugar. Sprinkle mixture on top of batter.
10. Bake at for 15 to 20 minutes or until golden brown.
11. Cool and cut into 8 squares.

Hummus for Spring Vegetables
Serves 4

Ingredients
>1 15-1/2 ounce can, reduced sodium, garbanzo beans, drained and rinsed
>1 tablespoon tahini
>2 tablespoons lemon juice
>2 cloves garlic, chopped
>1/4 teaspoon salt
>1/4 1/2 cup water (no more than 1/2 cup of water because you want a thick texture)
>1/4 cup parsley, chopped
>A pinch of cayenne pepper

Directions
1. Place beans in a processor or blender. Add the tahini, lemon juice, garlic, salt, and cayenne. Whiz until smooth.
2. Scrape into a bowl and stir in the parsley.
3. Serve with fresh cut up vegetables or as a sandwich spread.

Five Star Fruit Salad
Serves 6

Ingredients
>1 sweet pineapple, peeled, cored, and diced into small cubes
>1 mango, peeled and sliced into thin strips
>3 green Anjou pears, cored and diced into small cubes
>1 large ruby-red grapefruit, segmented
>Seeds of 1 pomegranate
>Juice of 5 limes
>3 tablespoons honey

Directions
1. Combine all fruit, or layer in a clear bowl.
2. Whip together the lime juice and honey.
3. Pour dressing on fruit.

Rice Pudding
Serves 5

Ingredients
6 cups water
2 cinnamon sticks
1 cup rice
3 cups skim milk
2/3 cup sugar
1/2 teaspoon salt

Directions
1. Put the water and cinnamon sticks into a medium saucepan. Bring to a boil.
2. Stir in rice. Cook on low heat for 30 minutes until rice is soft and water has evaporated.
3. Add skim milk, sugar and salt. Cook for another 15 minutes until it thickens.
4. Serve warm or cold.

Sweet Potato Custard
Serves 6

Ingredients
1 cup cooked mashed sweet potato
1/2 cup mashed banana (about 2 small bananas)
1 cup evaporated skim milk
2 tablespoons packed brown sugar
2 beaten egg yolks (or 1/3 cup egg substitute)
1/2 teaspoon salt
1/4 cup raisins
1 tablespoon sugar
1 teaspoon ground cinnamon
Non-stick spray coating

Directions
1. Preheat oven to 300° F.
2. In a medium bowl stir together sweet potato and banana.
3. Add milk, blending well.
4. Add brown sugar, egg yolks, and salt, mixing thoroughly.
5. Spray a 1 quart casserole with nonstick spray coating.
6. Transfer sweet potato mixture to casserole.
7. Combine raisins, sugar, and cinnamon; sprinkle over top of sweet potato mixture.
8. Bake in oven for 45 to 50 minutes or until a knife inserted near center comes out clean.

Coconut Macaroons
Serves 12

Ingredients
    1-1/4 cups sweetened flaked coconut
    1-1/2 cups crisped rice cereal
    2 egg whites
    3 tablespoons granulated sugar
    1 teaspoon vanilla extract
    1/8 teaspoon coconut extract

Directions
1. Preheat the oven to 300° F.
2. Line two baking sheets with parchment paper or spray with nonstick cooking spray.
3. In a medium baking pan or shallow baking dish, evenly spread the coconut in a thin layer.
4. Bake, stirring every 5 minutes, until lightly browned throughout, about 15 minutes.
5. Remove and let cool.
6. Raise the oven heat to 350° F.
7. In a medium bowl, combine the cooled coconut, rice cereal, egg whites, sugar, vanilla, and coconut extract; stir with a spatula until well combined.

8. Moisten your hands and shape the mixture into walnutsize balls, compacting the balls so they hold together.
9. Place on the prepared baking sheets.
10. Bake until lightly browned, about 20 minutes; cool at least 30 minutes on a rack before serving.

Watermelon Blueberry Banana Split
Serves 4

Ingredients
> 2 large bananas
> 8 scoops watermelon
> 2 cups fresh blueberries
> 1/2 cup vanilla low-fat yogurt
> 1/4 cup crunchy cereal nuggets

Directions
1. Peel bananas and cut in half crosswise, then cut each piece in half lengthwise.
2. For each serving, lay 2 banana pieces against the sides of a shallow dish.
3. Place a watermelon scoop at each end of the dish.
4. Fill the center space with the blueberries.
5. Stir yogurt until smooth. Spoon over the watermelon scoops.
6. Sprinkle with cereal nuggets.

Berry Delicious Pie
Serves 2

Ingredients
> 4-5 medium strawberries
> 1/4 cup raspberries
> 1 tablespoon + 1 teaspoon strawberry glaze (sugar free)
> 2 graham cracker crusts (individual size)
> Whipped topping (pressurized)

Directions
1. Wash strawberries and raspberries.
2. Remove stems from strawberries and cut into quarters.
3. Mix strawberry pieces and raspberries together in a bowl.
4. Chop until pieces are small.
5. Spread about 1 teaspoon of strawberry glaze on the bottom and sides of pie crust.
6. Add strawberry/raspberry mixture (about 2 tablespoons).
7. Top with 1 teaspoon of strawberry glaze.
8. Top with whipped topping as desired.
9. Serve immediately or place in refrigerator until ready to serve.

Baked Sliced Apples
Serves 4

Ingredients
>2 oranges
>2 tablespoons honey
>1/4 teaspoon ground cinnamon
>1/4 teaspoon ground cloves
>3 Granny Smith apples, peeled, cored and cut in 1/2 inch slices
>5 tablespoons raisins
>1/4 cup walnuts, chopped and divided
>1/4 cup low-fat vanilla yogurt

Directions
1. Preheat the oven to 500° F.
2. Grate the zest of one of the oranges and set aside.
3. Squeeze the juice form both oranges into a small bowl.
4. Stir the honey, cinnamon, cloves, and half the zest into the juice.
5. Lay half the apple slices in a glass baking dish.
6. Scatter the raisins and 2 tablespoons of the walnuts on top.
7. Pour on half the juice mixture and top with remaining apples and juice.

8. Combine the remaining 2 tablespoons walnuts with the orange zest and scatter over the top.
9. Cover lightly with foil and bake 30 minutes or until the apples are soft and the juices, bubbly.
10. Serve warm or cold with a dollop of low-fat vanilla yogurt.

Apple-Raisin Sauce
Serves 9

Ingredients
> 1-1/4 cups apple juice
> 1/2 cup apple butter
> 2 tablespoons molasses
> 1/2 cup raisins
> 1/4 teaspoon ground cinnamon
> 1/4 teaspoon ground nutmeg
> 1/2 teaspoon orange zest (optional)

Directions
1. Stir all ingredients together in medium saucepan.
2. Bring to a simmer over low heat. Let the sauce simmer 5 minutes.
3. Serve warm.

Bread Pudding
Serves 9

Ingredients
> 10 slices whole wheat bread
> 1 egg
> 3 egg whites
> 1-1/2 cups skim milk
> 1/4 cup sugar
> 1/4 cup brown sugar
> 1 teaspoon vanilla extract
> 1/2 teaspoon cinnamon
> 1/4 teaspoon nutmeg

1/4 teaspoon cloves
2 teaspoons sugar
Vegetable oil spray

Directions
1. Preheat the oven to 350° F.
2. Spray 8x8 inch baking dish with vegetable oil spray.
3. Lay slices of bread in the baking dish in two rows, overlapping them like shingles.
4. In a medium mixing bowl, beat together the egg, egg whites, milk, 1/4 cup sugar, the brown sugar, and vanilla.
5. Pour the egg mixture over the bread.
6. In a small bowl stir together the cinnamon, nutmeg, cloves, and sugar.
7. Bake the pudding for 30 to 35 minutes, until it has browned on top and is firm to the touch.
8. Serve warm or at room temperature, with warm apple raisin sauce.

I have high blood sugars, and Type 2 diabetes is not going to kill me. But I just have to eat right, and exercise, and lose weight, and watch what I eat, and I will be fine for the rest of my life. Tom Hanks